The Veterinary Assisting Essential Book of Knowledge

Companion Animals

This book is dedicated to my wonderfully supportive family for all of their assistance, guidance and understanding.

"Animals are such agreeable friends -
they ask no questions, they pass no
criticisms." ~ George Elliot

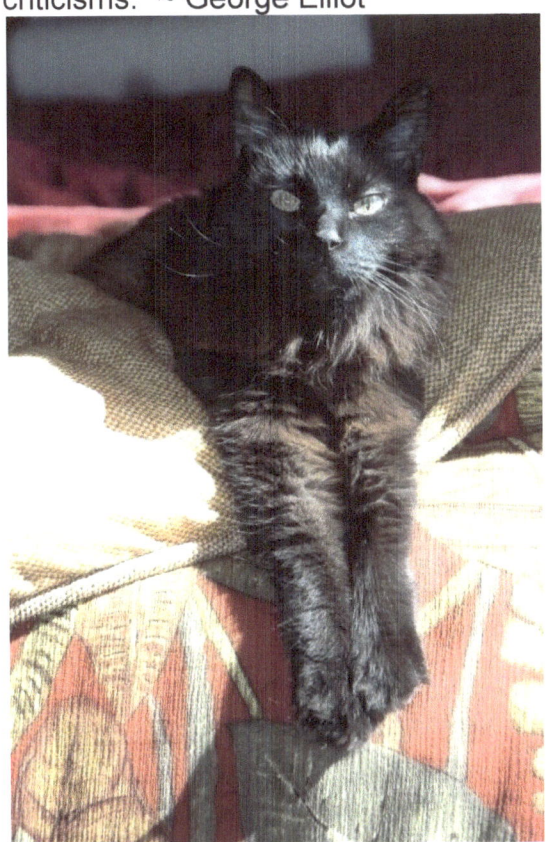

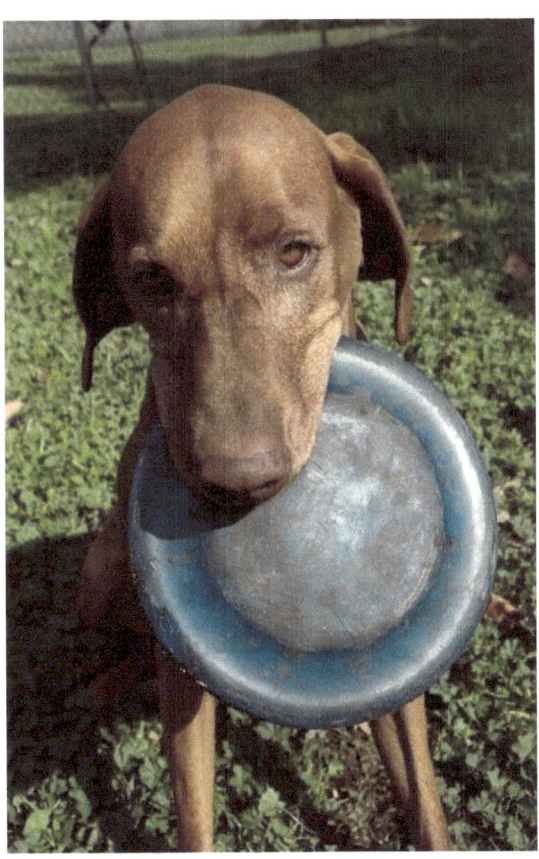

"All of the animals except for man know
that the principle business of life is to
enjoy it." ~ Samuel Butler

Table of Contents

Preface

I think I was like most boys; I was going to be a fireman, policeman or veterinarian. It probably had something to do with the sirens and uniforms, and for the latter, because of the animals. My father's hobby was falconry, so, I was always surrounded by animals of all kinds. His passion for animals was profound; his birds were beautiful, majestic and unique. I remember going hawking with him and witnessing the natural hunting struggle, both successes and failures that birds of prey go through to survive. I would eventually train and fly a kestrel and participate in many bird related research projects with my father.

With the promise of a well paying engineering job, my college focus began to move away from animal science; the emphasis was now on computer language, calculus and physics. After two years, it was obvious that engineering was not my passion.

My veterinary career started in a hardware store. A customer approached me looking for some tubing. He was a well dressed man, confident and courteous. I asked him what the tubing was to be used for and he said it was to be used on an anesthetic machine. He went on to tell me that he had just purchased a veterinary practice in town and was getting things ready for its opening. I began work as a veterinary assistant at Adobe Animal Hospital two weeks later. I learned all that I could as quickly as I could; it seemed so easy, so understandable and so rewarding. I had finally found my passion. Don was a great teacher and role model. He held very high standards for himself and I aspired to emulate his ethics. He allowed me to expand my skills as a veterinary assistant and technician.

Don is the most capable veterinarian I have worked with in my twenty-four year veterinary medicine career. In his office, he had, and still has, a binder with special procedures, drug doses and other important information; it is entitled 'the essential book of knowledge', and is the inspiration for this book. With this 'essential book of knowledge', my hope is that aspiring veterinary assistants, technicians or veterinarians are able to have a concise veterinary resource to refer to when needed. The Veterinary Assisting Essential Book of Knowledge covers the basics of veterinary medicine and concepts relating to companion animals (dogs and cats). I believe the key to veterinary medicine is confidence during animal restraint, injections or any aspect of the veterinary field. Take the information from these pages, build your confidence and aspire to be the best you can be.

My deepest gratitude goes to Don Wood, DVM, and his professional staff at Adobe Animal Hospital in Ramona, California, and my wonderful daughter, Rachel, for her exceptional illustrations.

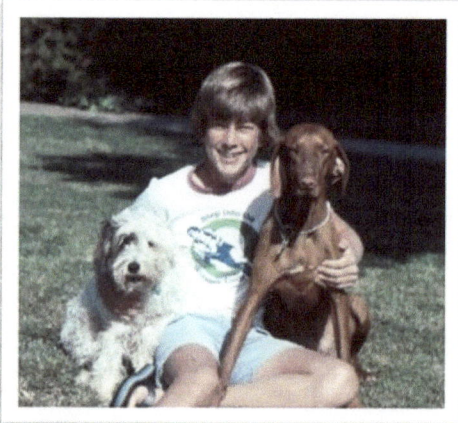

My first dog, Snuff (left), and Velvet

Introduction to Veterinary Medicine

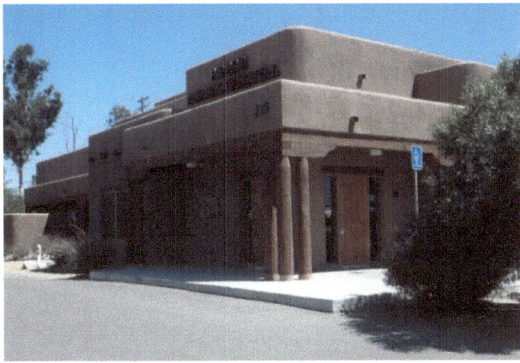

Figure 1: The modern veterinary practice

Veterinary medicine has a long history. The use of farm animals for work and food, as well as the domestication of companion animals, created a need for veterinary care and husbandry. The term 'veterinary' comes from the Latin word *Veterinae*, meaning 'of cattle or similar domestic animals'.

The Modern Veterinary Practice

The modern companion animal veterinary practice has many facets. The facility contains all the elements necessary to provide veterinary care to its patients. This includes areas for pet exams, treatment, radiology, dentistry, surgery and patient recovery. The modern veterinary clinic also serves as a pharmacy, as well as a pet boarding and grooming facility. Clients are greeted by a receptionist and are provided a waiting area for themselves and their pets. Some clinics have waiting areas that are segregated for dogs and cats. Some veterinary practices provide specialty and emergency care. These facilities specialize in surgery, oncology, ophthalmology, dermatology and critical care and in some cases are open twenty-four hours a day.

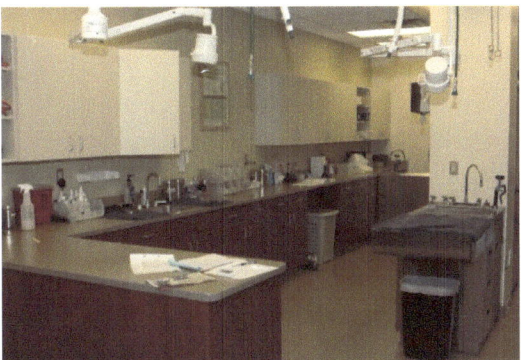

Figure 2: Treatment area

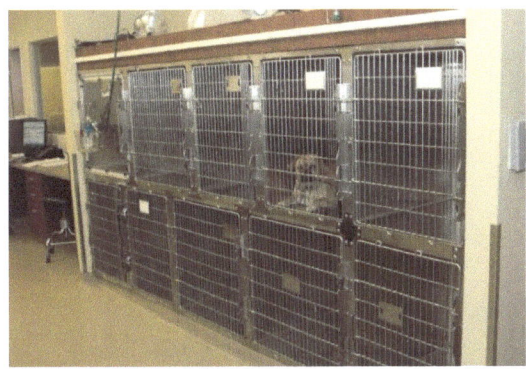

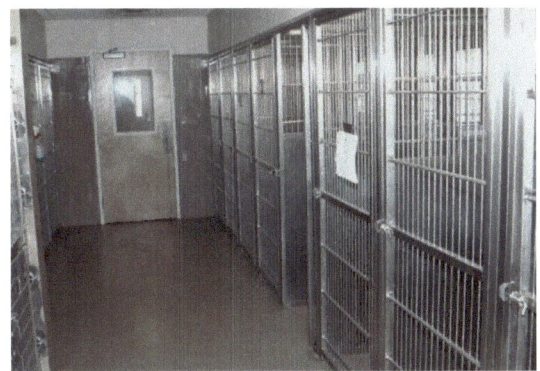

Figure 3: Animal recovery and holding cages

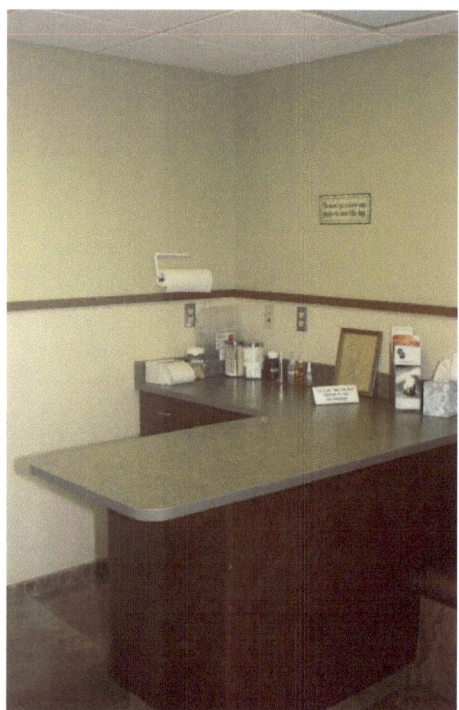
Figure 4: Patient examination room

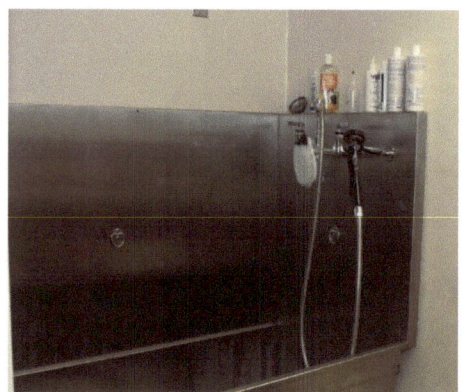
Figure 5: Pet bathing tub

The Modern Veterinary Team

The DVM
The root of all veterinary practices is the Doctor of Veterinary Medicine (DVM). This individual has obtained advanced college degrees in animal science. Many aspiring veterinarians first obtain a Bachelor's degree (BS) in Biology or another related field prior to applying to veterinary school. A Bachelor's degree can be obtained at most of the many four-year colleges in the country.

Following completion of the four-year undergraduate coursework related to veterinary medicine, an individual can apply to any of the 28 veterinary colleges in 26 North American states, as well as a multitude of international schools. Currently, there are over 700 veterinary schools worldwide. Graduates of a North America Veterinary College are then able to take a state or national veterinary exam to become a licensed veterinarian. International graduates must take additional testing prior to being licensed in the United States. The American Veterinary Medical Association (AVMA) regulates and gives accreditation to veterinary schools in the United States and abroad.

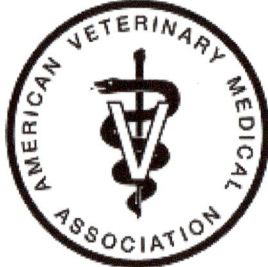

Currently, two veterinary schools can be found in California: UC Davis School of Veterinary Medicine (Sacramento) and Western University of Health Sciences (Pomona, Cal Poly).

The responsibilities given a licensed graduate of Veterinary Medicine include: diagnosis of disease, prescribing of medications and performing surgery. Additionally, veterinarians must adhere to the principles of veterinary medical ethics outlined by the AVMA. These ethics include, but are not limited to the following:

- Veterinarians should first consider the needs of the patient: to relieve disease, suffering, or disability while minimizing pain or fear.

- In emergencies, veterinarians have an ethical responsibility to provide essential services for animals, when necessary to save life or relieve suffering, subsequent to client agreement. Such emergency care may be limited to euthanasia to relieve suffering, or to stabilize the patient for transport to another source of animal care.
- Regardless of practice ownership, the interests of the patient, client and public require that all decisions that affect diagnosis, care, and treatment of patients are made by veterinarians.
- Veterinarians and their associates should protect the personal privacy of patients and clients.

(A complete list of ethics can be found at the AVMA website http://www.avma.org/issues/policy/ethics.asp)

The cost of obtaining a Doctorate in Veterinary Medicine can be expensive depending on schools attended, residency status and exam fees. It is estimated that in-state tuition for UC Davis would be approximately $180,000 for a four-year degree in veterinary medicine (2009).

The RVT

The Registered Veterinary Technician (RVT) is a licensed veterinary support individual who aids the veterinarian in the tasks of a veterinary practice. The RVT could be looked at as analogous to a Registered Nurse (RN) in human medicine. Just as with DVM's, Registered Veterinary Technicians must obtain advanced degrees and pass state exams in order to perform the duties of the RVT. Most aspiring RVT's attend an AVMA accredited school for animal health technology. After completion of the two-year coursework, the student is awarded an associate's degree in animal health technology. Part of the studies include on the job training, an essential component to learning the highly technical skills necessary for the RVT position. Graduates can then sit for the state exam required for licensing. There is also a national exam available to students who wish to be licensed in all states. This is an important consideration for those who might move to another state from where they obtained their degree.

Recently, several online programs have become available to aspiring Registered Veterinary Technicians. These programs give students the freedom to go at their own pace and enable them to balance education and employment effectively. They, however, tend to be more expensive than their traditional counterparts. These programs do require hands-on experience in a veterinary facility.

Some states recognize the value of on the job training and offer alternative programs to enable qualified persons the opportunity to take the RVT exam. This information can be found in the Veterinary Medical Board section of most states' consumer affairs website.

Ensure that your college or online program is AVMA accredited.

Under the supervision of a veterinarian, Registered Veterinary Technician responsibilities include nursing care, surgical assistance, laboratory sample collection and testing, radiology and client education. Furthermore, RVT's are licensed to perform the following tasks:

- Application of bandages and casts
- Anesthetic induction of patients
- Dental extractions
- Closure of surgical incisions
- Creation of punctures in skin for catheter placement

The RVT acronym is not universally utilized throughout the country. Other acronyms include:

- CVT -Certified Veterinary Technician
- LVT -Licensed Veterinary Technician
- AHT -Animal Health Technician

Additionally, some veterinary technicians specialize in specific areas of veterinary medicine, or obtain advanced degrees. These technicians may be referred to as Veterinary Technologists, or technician specialists.

The VA
The role of the veterinary assistant is one of assistant to the DVM and RVT. The job description for this entry level position includes animal handling and restraint, cleaning kennels and instruments, feeding and grooming animals, stocking supplies, office duties, as well as client interaction. Most veterinary assistants obtain on the job training and require little experience. Recently, there has been a move to certify veterinary assistants; this would enable candidates to meet skill requirements for the job description. The certification process would include an exam of competency. There are also online programs available for the aspiring veterinary assistant. These programs, like online RVT programs, tend to be more expensive, but enable students to proceed at their own pace.

Many states provide vocational education in the form of a regional occupational program (ROP), or career and technical education (CTE). These programs provide tuition-free job skills in many industries including veterinary assisting. Classes are provided to interested students ages sixteen and older. The ROP veterinary assisting program usually includes hands on work and on the job training.

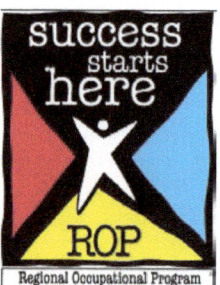

The Receptionist
The primary role of the veterinary receptionist is client interaction. The receptionist is usually responsible for admitting and discharging patients, communicating with clients in the waiting room or on the phone, collecting fees, scheduling appointments and filing records. As most medical and veterinary facilities move toward electronic medical record systems, the receptionists of the future will need greater computer skills.

The first and last person the client sees and has interaction with, is the receptionist.

Other Veterinary Related Careers

Veterinary professionals and support staff can be found in many other areas of veterinary medicine. Areas such as research, academics, grooming, boarding, drug companies, welfare and law enforcement, pet food and supply companies and laboratories, offer employment opportunities for individuals interested in veterinary medicine. Although many of these areas don't work with animals directly, they require a good working understanding and background in animal health and medicine.

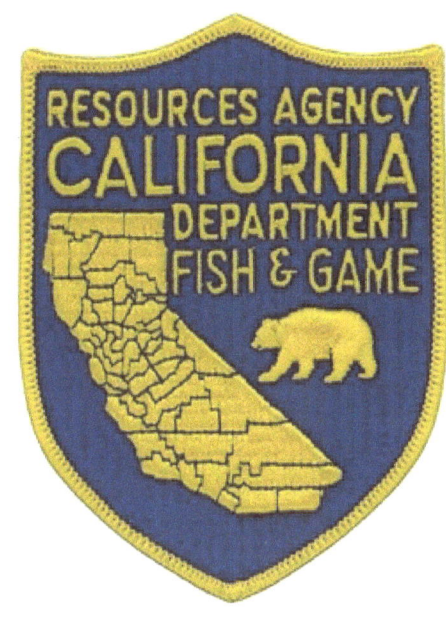

Overview of Law

The Department of Consumer Affairs is designed to protect and serve consumers while ensuring a competent and fair marketplace. Furthermore, it regulates licensing of many industries including veterinary professionals. The Veterinary Medical Board oversees many of the issues relating to veterinarians and veterinary practices. State laws vary, so determining current laws applicable to veterinary medicine in one's state of practice should be researched periodically.

Laws Governing Job Duties

By law, the following duties can only be performed by a licensed veterinarian (DVM):

- Diagnose disease
- Perform surgery
- Prescribe medications

By law, the following duties can only be performed by a DVM or Registered Veterinary Technician (RVT):

- Induce anesthesia
- Perform dental extractions
- Close existing wounds
- Apply bandages and splints
- Make a puncture in skin to place a catheter

The RVT can perform these tasks under direct or indirect supervision. These tasks are specific to California and may vary slightly in other states.

By law, a veterinary assistant (VA) can perform any but the above duties under direct or indirect supervision of a DVM or under direct supervision of a RVT. These duties may include giving injections, surgical assistance, radiography, phlebotomy, dental prophylaxis, and laboratory testing among others.

Direct supervision means that the DVM is within the veterinary premises and is quickly and easily available. Indirect supervision means the veterinarian is not in the premises, but has left detailed instructions regarding the care to be given. In both cases, the veterinarian has previously examined the animal.

Animal care and welfare organizations are in place to help animals of all types. Animal welfare law enforcement can be managed by local police departments as well as animal control facilities. Some Humane Societies provide animal enforcement services. These services include management of stray dogs, injured dogs, cats, wildlife, noise issues, animal attacks, as well as neglect cases. The Department of Fish and Game regulates wildlife, hunting regulations and possession of wild animals.

Several non-profit organizations provide services for injured and orphaned animals and are outspoken proponents of wildlife care, compassion and animal rights. These organizations include the People for the Ethical Treatment of Animals (PETA), Greenpeace, the Fund for Animals and Project Wildlife.

Animal Rights Laws

Animal rights laws are in place in order to ensure minimum standards of animal welfare are met. Some of the laws include the following:

- Sanitation
  - Animals are required to have sanitary living conditions, food and water.
- Emergency treatment
  - Most states provide the ability for animals to receive medical care in

cases of emergency. This law protects the Good Samaritan from incurring costs related to the emergency treatment. State animal control would reimburse the clinic for the care and search for the legal owner once the pet is stable.

- Euthanasia can be legally performed on an animal at any time. Most cases involve medical conditions, but some are necessary due to aggression and biting. Owners have the right to euthanize their pet for any reason as long as the pet has not bitten anyone within ten days.
- The California abandonment law enables veterinarians to relocate or humanely euthanize animals abandoned at a veterinary practice. Other states may have similar laws to protect practitioners from the burden of abandoned pets.

Animal Care Laws

- Leash law
  - Many states have laws ensuring animals are restrained by a six foot leash when in public places.
- Nuisance
  - Nuisance laws provide recourse for individuals living in proximity to animals causing public disturbances. Animal barking and howling are among the most common reasons for this law.
- Neglect

  - Most state provide for punishment to individuals who neglect and don't properly care for an animal. These laws are generally enforced by state animal control officers.
- Wildlife
  - By law, most wildlife is protected from possession or harassment. Special permits are required to possess wildlife and rehabilitation organizations must also have special handling permits.
- Animal licensing laws
  - Dogs must be vaccinated against rabies virus at 4 months of age, or within 1 month of their acquisition. Most states require rabies vaccination and licensing of all dogs; vaccines are given annually or every three years. States charge fees to license one's pets.
  - Cats are not currently required, by law, to be vaccinated against rabies virus; they are not required to be licensed. It is encouraged to vaccinate all pets against this deadly zoonotic disease.

Dogs are required by law to be vaccinated against Rabies virus.

Veterinary premise laws include several important documentation requirements. Medical records and radiographs are considered the property of the veterinary clinic and are also considered 'legal documents'. For this reason, medical record information must be properly recorded and maintained. Here are some important requirements:

- Entries in medical records should be made in pen only; pencil is considered unacceptable because entries could be tampered with or erased.
- 'White out' should never be used in a medical record. If changes are needed, a single line crossing out the entry is the acceptable method.
- Medical records and radiographs must be kept for 3 years after the client's last visit, or if the pet is deceased. This timeline may vary in some states.

In addition to medical record requirements, veterinary clinics must maintain detailed records (logs) of the following:

- Anesthesia log
  - Provides patient information, anesthetics used and type and duration of the procedure.
- Radiology exposure log
  - Provides patient information, x-ray exposure techniques, number of radiographs taken and person taking radiographs.
- Controlled drug log
  - Provides patient information, quantity of controlled drug dispensed and balance of drug remaining in stock.

Electronic medical records are undoubtedly changing the way medical records are kept and maintained. Computer based record systems allow for easier information transfer and storage. Medical cases can be shared with consultants and specialists electronically, saving time and money. Digital radiographs can be sent to other clinics or specialists by the same method as electronic medical records.

Controlled Drug Log Diazepam 5mg			
Date	**Patient**	**Quantity Dispensed**	**Balance** 100
8/1/11	Bruzer	20	80
8/4/11	Skeeter	32	48

Table 1: Generic Controlled Drug Log

Importance of Health and Safety in Veterinary Medicine

Workplace safety is an important facet of any occupation. Worker injuries not only hurt the individual, but affect others when an individual is away from work. Workplace injury and workers compensation costs billions of dollars annually. Small businesses can be particularly affected. Prevention is essential to the livelihood of many veterinary practices that lack additional staff to replace an injured worker. In addition to structured health and safety programs, businesses must adhere to guidelines set by the Occupational Safety and Health Administration (OSHA). OSHA's mission is 'To ensure safe and healthful working conditions for working men and women by setting and enforcing standards and by providing training, outreach, education, and assistance.' Violations can result in significant fines. Veterinary health and safety includes office safety, but additionally, animal, radiation, anesthesia and zoonotic disease concerns.

Office Safety Issues and Considerations

Fire extinguishers
- Know their locations and how to use them.

Cabinets
- Be careful not to overweight upper shelves of pull-out cabinets or leave them open.

Spills
- Clean up any spill immediately. Use cones or placard to caution others of slippery floors.

Office supplies
- Use sharp items such as utility knifes and staplers with caution.

Break room
- Maintain break room cleanliness for both esthetics and sanitary reasons. Wash your hands before eating.

Electrical
- Don't overload electrical outlets and circuits.

Ergonomics with computers/work stations
- Use proper chair height, computer height and distance from monitor.

Posture
- Be aware of good posture to reduce back and muscle fatigue. Leaning over exam tables can put significant strain on your back.

Lifting objects
- Use proper lifting techniques when lifting office supplies such as boxes or bulky items; bend at the knees, not at the back.

Veterinary Medicine Safety Issues and Considerations

Animal Related Injuries and Hazards

Traumatic injuries are a way of life in veterinary medicine. Animals can be unpredictable and in some situations may behave uncharacteristically. Painful injuries or procedures may cause a normally friendly animal to become aggressive. It is imperative that the veterinary team recognizes animal behavior types as well as utilizes animal restraint equipment in order to reduce personnel injury. Of the 74.8 million dogs in the United States, dogs account

for most bites, 4.5 million annually. Seventy percent of these animals belong to the victim's family or a friend. In 2010, thirty-four fatalities were reported from dog bites. (dogbitelaw.com)
Both dog and cat bites can lead to serious injury and infection, so prevention is paramount. Cat bites, however, can cause infection in up to eighty percent of their victims. This is compared to three to eighteen percent infection producing bites from dogs. (vetmed.lsu.edu). In order to understand why this occurs, one needs to take a closer look at the dental anatomy of dogs and cats.

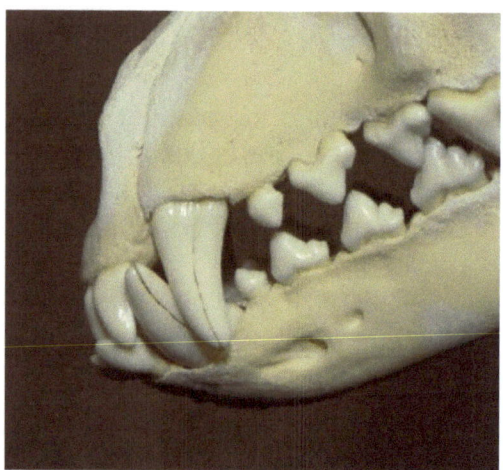
Figure 6: Dog teeth produce a blunt crushing bite

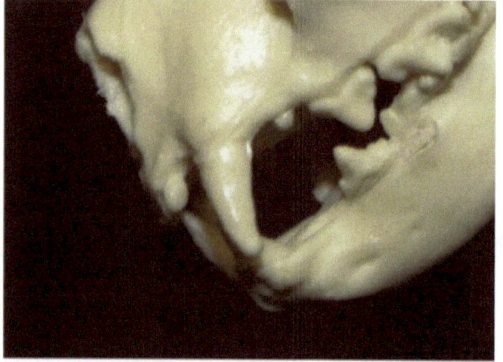
Figure 7: Cat teeth produce a small pointed bite

Scratches can be common and also lead to serious injury to the veterinary team. Cat scratch fever, a bacterial

You are more likely to get an infection from a cat bite.

disease, is transmitted by cat scratches and bites and can lead to localized inflammation at the site of infection. Usually not serious, most cat scratches can be minimally or moderately painful to the victim.

Prevention of both bites and scratches by small animals can be facilitated with several different kinds of restraint and control devices.

Dog and cat muzzles are an easy way to reduce animal bites in a veterinary practice. Popular muzzles are made of nylon or mesh, and act to prevent an animal from opening its mouth while allowing for the ability to breath. Basket muzzles allow the pet to open its mouth during times of respiratory distress. Most muzzles have a nylon neck strap with easy snap closure. Muzzles should be carefully applied over the snout of the animal and then secured behind the head with the neck strap. Once placed, some animals may try and remove the muzzle with their feet; preventing this will ensure the muzzle stays secure. Cat muzzles are designed to cover the pet's snout, as well as cover their eyes. Doing so has a calming effect on most cats as well as minimizing their ability to target a bite. A muzzle can also be fashioned from a piece of conforming bandage material. Make a loop with the bandage material, place over the pet's snout, then secure around the back of their head.

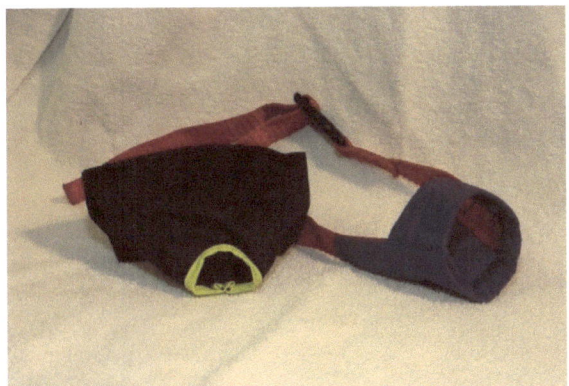

Leashes are another effective means of pet restraint in a veterinary practice. A choke style leash is less likely to be removed by the pet under adverse situations. Leashes should be placed on both dogs and cats while the pets are in the veterinary practice and are not secure in a cage. A leash can prevent an animal from escaping and potentially injuring itself or others. A leash can be threaded through a fence or eyelet on the wall to further secure a pet; this secures the animals head and neck, while enabling access to the rest of the pet's body.

Gauntlet and welding gloves are usually made of a heavy fabric or leather and are effective in protecting the hands and forearms of an animal restrainer. Many bites cannot penetrate the heavy material, but the glove does not eliminate the possibility of being bitten. These heavy gloves, though protective, reduce the animal restrainer's ability to hold an animal as tightly as when using one's hands alone.

Sedatives can be used to calm or immobilize an animal if other means are not feasible or are unsafe for both the animal and handler. Sedatives are generally given to a pet, orally, or by injection. Many feral cats and dogs require sedatives before they can be safely examined.

Other Veterinary Workplace Hazards

Allergic reactions to animal hair, dander and saliva are possible in hypersensitive individuals. Local skin redness, rashes, or bumps as well as nasal and ocular inflammation are common symptoms of an allergic reaction. The use of masks, eye protection and protective clothing can significantly reduce allergic reactions from pets.

It is essential to use proper lifting techniques when picking up and carrying pets. Always bend at the knees when lifting an animal up from the ground; avoid bending over the pet. Some animals are quite large and require assistance when being lifted. Two or more people may be required to lift a large Mastiff or Great Dane. Additionally, animals may attempt to move while being lifted, making back strain and twisting a serious problem.

Zoonoses or zoonotic diseases are defined as any disease that an animal can transmit to a person (Merck Veterinary manual). The World Health Organization reports that there are over 200 known Zoonoses worldwide. Types of zoonotic infectious agents include:
- Bacteria
- Parasites
- Viruses
- Fungi
- Prions

Transmission can occur as a result of a multitude of situations including contact with contaminated water, soil, fecal material, bodily fluids, or by a bite or scratch from an infected animal. A host is defined as an organism that harbors an infectious agent. Zoonotic diseases may be transmitted to the host by insects or other organisms; these intermediate organisms are called vectors. Gloves, face shields, masks and protective clothing are effective means of reducing exposure to potential Zoonoses. Furthermore, infectious disease screening and lab tests can identify animals with Zoonotic diseases.

A zoonotic disease is any disease transmitted from an animal to a person.

ZOONOTIC DISEASES

	Source Animals	Transmission/Vector	Human Symptoms
BACTERIAL DISEASES			
Anthrax	cattle, sheep, horse	skin, inhalation	septicemia of SQ lesions, URI
Brucellosis	cattle, dogs, sheep	placental contact, birth fluids	septicemia, flu-like symptoms
Campylobacteriosis	dog, cat, cattle	fecal, oral	gastroenteritis, diarrhea
Cat scratch disease	cat	bite, scratch, broken skin	fever, skin redness
Leptospirosis	dog, cat, rodent	urine, tissues	jaundice, bleeding, fever, muscle pain
Lyme disease	dog, deer, rodent	tick bite	anorexia, lethargy, lameness
Ornithosis(psittacosis)	bird	inhalation	URI, pneumonia
Pasteurellosis	cat, dog	bite wound	cellulites, septicemia
Rat-bite fevers	rodent	bite wound	systemic, febrile, polyarthritis
Rocky Mountain Spotted Fever	dog	tick bite	fever, headache, muscle pain, bleeding
Salmonellosis	mammal, bird, reptile	fecal, oral	gastroenteritis
Tetanus	mammal	puncture, bite	headache, fever, muscle spasms
Tuberculosis	mammal, bird	inhalation, ingestion	listlessness, chest pain, lung problems
FUNGAL DISEASES			
Cryptococcosis	bird (indirect)	inhalation	pneumonia-like
Ringworm (dermatophytosis)	mammal	direct contact	ring-like lesion of the skin, hair, nails
PARASITIC DISEASES			
Cryptosporidiosis	cattle	fecal-oral	gastroenteritis
Giardiasis	dog, cat,	fecal, water-oral	diarrhea, nausea, abdominal pain
Hookworm	dog, cat	direct contact	skin irritation
Roundworm	dog, cat	fecal-oral	systemic, blindness
Scabies (Sarcoptes)	dog, cat	direct contact	skin irritation, hair loss
Tapeworm	dog, cat, sheep, cattle	ingestion of flea	systemic, death
Toxoplasmosis	cat	fecal-oral	systemic, encephalitis
VIRAL DISEASES			
Herpesvirus simiae (B)	old world primates (macaques)	bite, scratch, mucous membranes, needle stick	meningioencephalitis, death
Newcastle disease	poultry	contact with eyes, aerosol	conjunctivitis, influenza
Rabies	warm blooded animals	saliva, bite	CNS signs, encephalomyelitis, death
West Nile Virus	mammal, bird	mosquito bite	fever, headache, rash
PRION DISEASE			
(BSE) Mad Cow Disease	cattle	Ingestion of contaminated meat or brain tissue	CNS signs, depression, dementia, difficulty walking

Syringes and needles are widely used in veterinary practices. An inadvertent needle puncture can lead to a vaccination or other drug self-inoculation. The effects depend on the drug inoculated, but may include local skin irritation, redness, or possibly anaphylaxis. Anaphylaxis is an acute, potentially life threatening allergic reaction to a chemical.

Prevention of drug self-inoculation involves the safe handling and use of syringes and needles. Recapping of needles should be discouraged, but if necessary, a 'no hand' recapping technique should be used. The needle cap is placed on a surface and the needle is re-capped without holding the cap. This ensures that an inadvertent needle stick to the hand holding the cap does not occur. Once the needle is placed partly into the cap, the syringe, needle, and cap can be rotated up allowing the needle to be capped into place.

Figure 9: Hands free needle re-capping technique

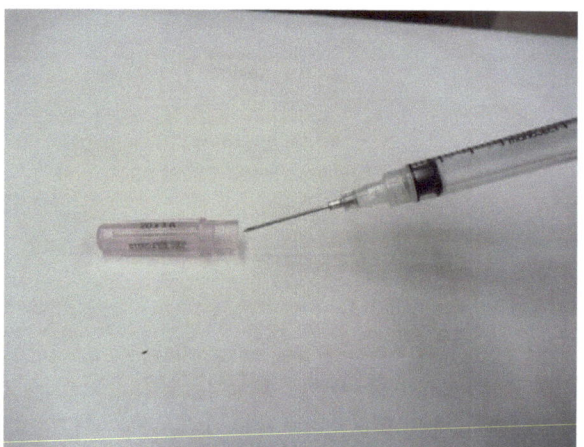

Step 1: Without holding cap, place needle in cap

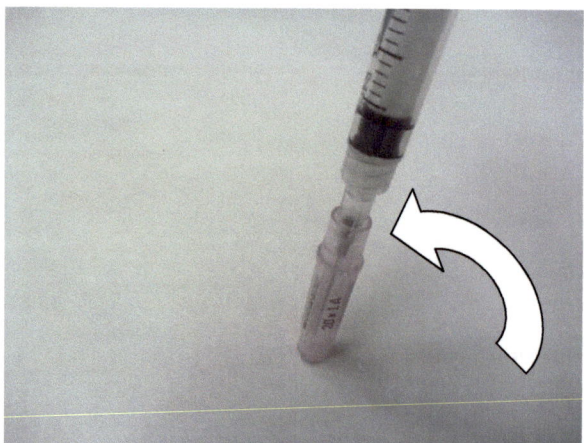

Step 2: Rotate syringe upwards and cap needle

Laboratory hazards primarily involve working with potentially infectious laboratory samples. These samples include animal feces, urine, blood, cultures and tissues. Exposure is usually by direct contact, inhalation, or ingestion. Prevention includes the use of gloves, masks, goggles, as well as laboratory ventilation hoods. Additionally, no eating or drinking should be allowed in work areas and hands should be washed frequently.

Gas anesthetics are frequently used in veterinary medicine. Their use enables the veterinary team to perform routine surgical procedures safely. Gas anesthetics like isoflurane, sevoflurane, and desflurane are safe and effective means in which to maintain a patient under anesthesia; however, there are potential hazards to the veterinary team. Exposure to anesthetic gases is usually caused by two means:

- Exposure to gases from the machine
- Exposure to waste gases from the patient

Gas anesthetics are liquids that evaporate into the gaseous state in the presence of air or heat. Filling of the anesthetic vaporizer can lead to spills and exposure of gaseous anesthetics.

Anesthetic machine circuit leaks can be an additional source of anesthetic gas exposure. Proper vaporizer filling techniques and anesthetic machine leak testing prior to use will reduce the possibility of anesthetic gas exposure. Furthermore, anesthetic gas scavenging systems, as well as proper room ventilation are effective ways to reduce exposure. A properly trained veterinary anesthetist should evaluate the anesthetic machine prior to every procedure. The use of a patient endotracheal tube reduces anesthetic gas leakage by over fifty percent when compared with an anesthetic mask. Waste gases are those eliminated or not utilized by the patient. Waste anesthetic gases are either redistributed in the patient circuit or removed by the anesthetic machine scavenging system. Once the patient is disconnected from the anesthetic machine, waste gasses are expelled into the patient's surrounding environment. Care must be taken to provide adequate ventilation in patient recovery areas, as well as minimize time spent near the patient's head and mouth.

Symptoms of gas anesthetic exposure include sedation, drowsiness, fatigue and headaches.

> **Anesthetic gases have distinctive odors that are easily identifiable.**

Non-anesthetic chemical hazards include pesticides, disinfectants, bleach, mercury, formaldehyde, baths, dips and assorted sprays. Exposure can occur from direct contact, ingestion, or inhalation. Protective gloves and safety goggles can prevent accidental exposure to these chemicals.

Example: DMSO (dimethyl sulfoxide) easily permeates the skin.

Compressed gases sometimes used in a veterinary practice include nitrogen, oxygen, carbon dioxide and nitrous oxide. These gases can be potentially flammable, combustible, or even explosive. Furthermore, compressed gas tanks, when not properly secured, could possibly fall, dislodging the valve and creating a gas driven torpedo-like projectile.

Radiation hazards in a veterinary practice are associated with the use of ionizing radiation called x-rays. The veterinarian uses this type of radiation to produce radiographic images of patients. X-ray radiation is not within the visible spectrum of light and therefore cannot be seen. It has the ability to penetrate the body easily, but is attenuated by metals such as lead. Exposure to x-ray radiation can cause cell damage and mutation, erythema (redness), abortion and fetal defects.

Dosimeters are used to monitor occupational radiation exposure. These small x-ray film badges are worn by the veterinary radiologist when taking x-rays. Periodically, exposure measurements are evaluated; several companies provide this fee-based service to veterinary professionals.

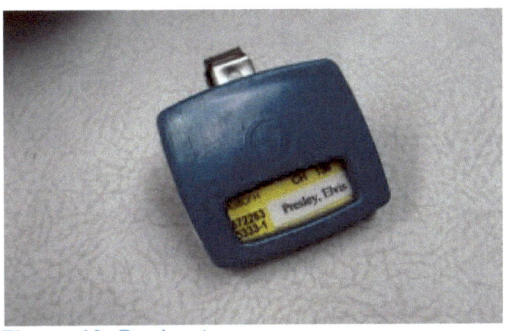

Figure 10: Dosimeter

Protection from direct x-ray exposure remains as the most effective means of radiation safety. Protection is facilitated by the following means:

- Time
- Distance
- Shielding

Reduction of time of exposure or number of exposures reduces one's occupational exposure to radiation. Just like a camera, adjustments to machine settings can reduce exposure time and produce a comparable image. By optimizing technique and patient positioning, one can also reduce the number of exposures necessary to obtain a diagnostic image.

Increased distance from primary x-ray beam can significantly reduce one's exposure to radiation. The use of restraint devices further helps reduce the need to be in close proximity to the primary beam.

The use of lead aprons, gloves and thyroid protectors helps shield one from x-ray exposure. Use of lead protective attire is imperative when restraining an animal on the x-ray table while an image is being taken. Lead gloves can be cumbersome and make animal restraint while taking radiographs more challenging. Lead barriers and walls also provide protection when animal restraint is not needed.

Traditional film processors containing chemical developers and fixers are being replaced with digital x-ray systems. These processors and chemicals can produce glutaraldehyde gas which can cause severe headaches in sensitive individuals. Proper ventilation is necessary when working with chemical film processors.

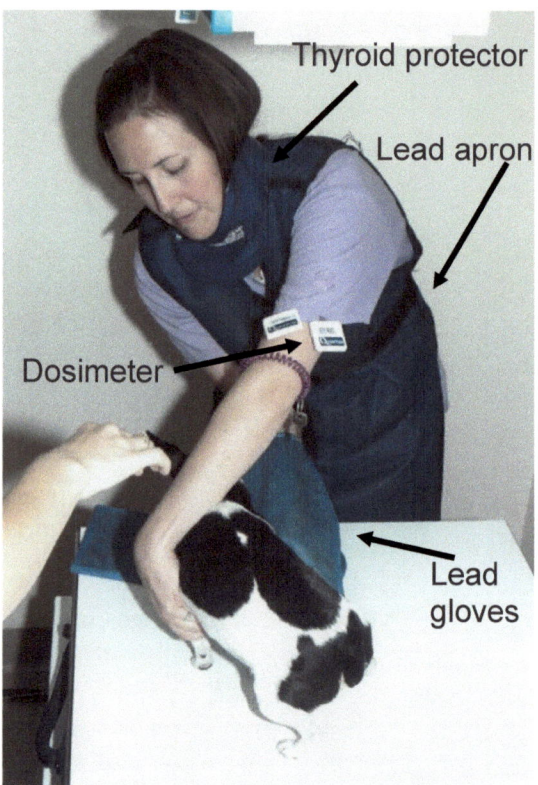

Figure 11: Radiation protective shielding and monitor

Note: Individuals under 18 years of age or pregnant are not allowed to take x-rays in a veterinary practice.

Medical wastes are waste materials generated in a health care facility. Medical wastes can be further classified by their specific type.

- Regulated bio-hazardous waste
  - Potentially zoonotic infectious wastes that includes tissues, blood and culture plates
- Regulated sharps waste
  - Needles, scalpel blades, glass microscope slides
- Medical solid waste

- o Surgical gloves, drapes, bandages, organs and tissues
- Medical liquid waste
  - o Body fluids, liquid blood, urine and non-hazardous fluids

Disposal of bio-hazardous and sharps waste is regulated by most local and state governments. This waste must be treated by a steam autoclave or disposed of by a registered hauler. Incineration and gel containment are common methods of regulated medical waste disposal. Veterinary non-contaminated medical solid waste can be disposed of in regular trash and medical liquid waste can be placed in a sanitary sewer system.

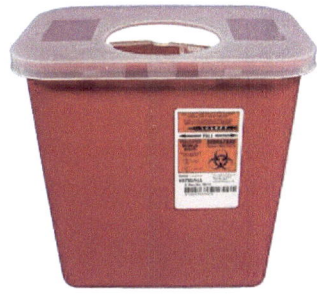

Figure 12: Sharps container

Material Safety Data Sheets (MSDS) are provided by manufacturers of chemicals and substances. These forms supply information on the properties and safe handling of workplace substances. Information includes physical properties, melting and flash points, toxicity, reactivity, health effects and first aid. A 'hard copy' of all data sheets should be found in a readily available location in a veterinary clinic; they should identify all products used there.

Reactivity placards should be placed on any chemical storage areas and on secondary containers containing substances. Numbers 0-4 are placed in the four colored squares indicating the severity of hazard. The reactivity scale is as follows:

4=Severe Hazard
3=Serious Hazard
2=Moderate Hazard
1=Slight Hazard
0=Minimal Hazard

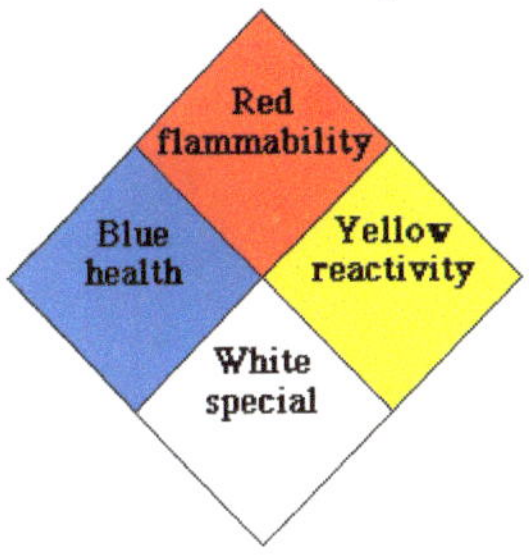

Figure 13: Reactivity Placard, and Hazard Scale

Hygiene is an important aspect of veterinary safety. Working with animals can be strenuous and lead to filthy attire. Medical smocks are rugged and can tolerate the demands of animal handling; improper attire can become damaged or torn. Jewelry such as looped earrings can become hooked or traumatically removed by a struggling pet. Long hair can get entangled if not properly secured. Following dress codes and appropriate attire is the best way to avoid hygiene injuries.

The bottom line with safety:
- Utilize proper equipment for the job.
- Use gloves, eye protection and proper uniforms.
- Get training in the use of chemicals and equipment.
- Ensure that equipment is in good working condition.
- No food or drink in work areas.
- Utilize proper ventilation.
- Wash hands regularly.

Sanitation

Sanitary working conditions are essential for the veterinary staff as well as for the health and safety of the clinics patients. Disease transmission can be greatly reduced by proper cleaning of the veterinary practice. By using antimicrobial cleaning products that inhibit the growth of microorganisms such as bacteria, fungi and protozoan's, nosocomial infections can be reduced. Nosocomial infections are those acquired in the hospital, and can be disastrous for the sick or immune compromised patient.

Sanitation can be broken down into two key elements: things that clean inanimate objects and things that clean living tissues. Disinfection is the process by which inanimate objects such as workspaces, countertops, floors, and animal housing are cleaned. Chemicals used to facilitate this usually have bactericidal, fungicidal and viricidal properties. These cleaning products, known as disinfectants, can contain some of the following components:

- Phenols
- Quaternary ammonium
- Aldehydes
- Sodium hypochlorite

Phenols are active ingredients in some household disinfectants. They can also be found in mouthwash and some hand soaps. Phenols can be corrosive to the skin and toxic to some individuals. SynPhenol, Lysol, and Environ are examples of phenol containing disinfectants used in some veterinary practices.

Quaternary ammonium products or 'quats' have disinfecting properties like phenols; however, they tend to be less effective when used with certain types of soaps. Examples used in veterinary practices include MintQuat and Roccal. *Aldehydes* such as formaldehyde and glutaraldehyde are very effective microbial killing agents. Formaldehyde can be useful as a disinfectant, but should be used carefully due to its carcinogenic effects. Glutaraldehyde is often used as a cold sterilization solution for instruments and endoscopes. Glutaraldehyde can irritate the eyes, skin and respiratory tract in some people and should be used in a well ventilated area.

Sodium hypochlorite is a useful and inexpensive disinfectant. Also known as bleach, it acts to oxidize the cell membranes of microorganisms; thus, destroying them. Organic material inhibits the activity of sodium hypochlorite; therefore, diligent cleaning of instruments and surfaces should take place prior to its use. Sodium hypochlorite readily inactivates in the presence of heat or sunlight; it can also bleach colors from clothing.

Antiseptics are cleaning products used on living tissue to reduce the possibility of infection. These products use components that are less harsh on sensitive skin and tissues. Antiseptics are commonly used to clean wounds and play an important role in surgical preparation. Some commonly used antiseptics include:

- Iodine
- Biguanidines
- Peroxide
- Alcohol

Iodine-containing antiseptics such as povidone-iodine (betadine) have effective antimicrobial properties. Furthermore, iodine offers residual properties that afford a persistent affect once applied; this is especially important for surgical preparation. Iodine containing products are brownish in color and when used may cause staining.

Biguanidines like chlorhexadine (Nolvasan, Hibiclens) are commonly used antiseptic solutions and soaps. Diluted solutions can be used for wound flushing and soaking, while soaps are generally used in surgical preparation. Chlorhexadine is also found in some mouthwash and is used to treat gingivitis.

Peroxide can be used as an antiseptic, but other products may afford superior antimicrobial benefits. Peroxide is still used to clean residual blood from tissues and fur and is useful in loosening debris in and around wounds.

Alcohol is an antiseptic used for injection site preparation, or in conjunction with an antiseptic soap for surgical site preparation. Alcohol can serve as a solvent to carry away debris. Care must be taken when using alcohol near the eyes or in open wounds, as its use can cause a painful burning sensation in these areas. Seventy percent isopropyl alcohol is one of the most commonly used alcohols in veterinary medicine.

> **Disinfectants are used on inanimate objects and surfaces, while antiseptics are used on living tissue.**

Cleaning Techniques

Countertops, floors, animal cages, veterinary equipment and instruments require cleaning and disinfection. The key to cleaning is 'contact time'. Allowing a disinfectant to stay on a surface for several minutes is better than immediately wiping it off. Soaking of equipment and instruments will allow for increased contact time and superior cleaning. Disinfectants in spray bottles allow a fine mist to be applied to virtually any area or surface. Mopping floors with disinfectant treated water is common and convenient. Animal cages should be cleaned from top to bottom; clean from less dirty area to most soiled area. This will allow for increased contact time on those surfaces that are more likely to be contaminated with urine and feces. It is also important to clean any cage doors, as these surfaces, though less easy to clean, can be contaminated as well.

All surfaces of instruments, including joint surfaces, should be cleaned of all organic material. A mildly abrasive cleaning brush and soap helps with the cleaning process. Soaking or ultrasonic cleaning of instruments will dislodge dried blood and material otherwise difficult to remove by conventional methods. All instruments, especially those with hinges and moving parts, should be immersed in an instrument milk or lubricating protectant and allowed to dry after being thoroughly cleaned.

Aseptic surgical site preparation is an important aspect of veterinary surgery. The technique employs the concept of contact time and use of antiseptics to produce a 'sterile field' for a multitude of surgeries. A common method of surgical preparation is termed 'triple prep', where the surgical site is cleaned with antiseptic soap and alcohol at least three times before considering the site 'sterile'. Antiseptic soap-soaked gauze sponges are useful for the initial cleaning of the surgical site. Here is the process:

1. Working from the inside of the surgical area, apply the soaked gauze sponges to the skin and scrub towards the outer perimeter. In doing so, dirt and debris will be worked away from the surgical field. Remember, contact time is an important part of the cleaning process.
2. An alcohol soaked gauze sponge can then be used to remove the soap from the surgical field in the same manner as the soap was applied.
3. Process 1 and 2 are repeated at least three times or until no dirt residue remains on any of the sponges.
4. Use of a betadine or chlorhexadine 'top coat' is beneficial in inhibiting bacterial growth during surgery.

Once the top coat has been applied, the surgical area should be considered sterile and care should be taken not to contaminate the site.

> **'Contact time' is important when cleaning living and non-living surfaces.**

Sterilization Techniques

Sterilization is designed to kill all living things, and therefore, living animals cannot be completely sterilized. We look at the sterile field created on an animal as a surface as clean as possible, devoid of as many microorganisms as possible. Surgical equipment and instruments, however, can be completely sterilized. Many sterilization processes are available and used in the veterinary practice.

Cold sterilization is the process where instruments are stored in a tray and are immersed in a powerful chemical disinfectant. These instruments are used for minor medical procedures where surgical sterilization is not necessary. Solusterile, Cidex and chlorhexadine are commonly used cold sterilization solutions. These solutions should be changed on a frequent basis; especially once the cold sterilization tray has been used for a procedure and is potentially contaminated.

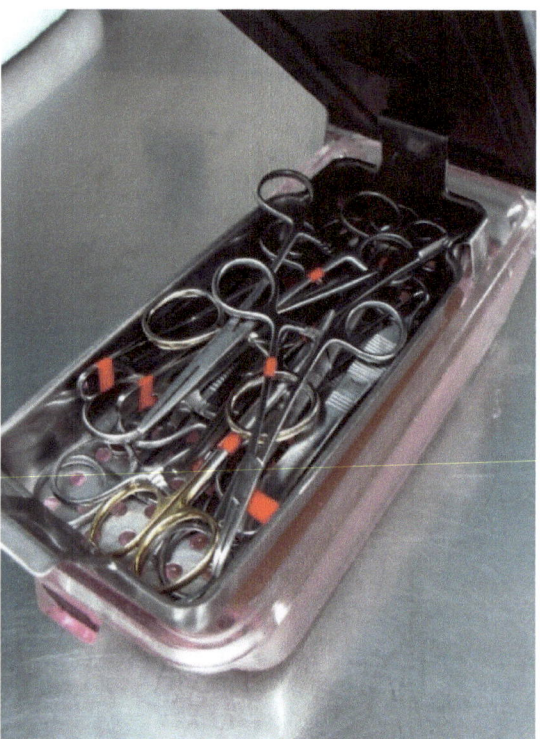

Figure 14: Cold sterilizer and instruments

Steam autoclaves are the most common means by which instruments and equipment are surgically sterilized in veterinary practices. Much like a kitchen pressure cooker, steam autoclaves utilize heated steam under pressure to generate temperatures and penetrability necessary to kill microorganisms in and on surgical equipment. Cloth drapes, gowns and towels, metal instruments and durable plastics can be sterilized using this method. Because of the high temperatures generated in a short period, steam autoclave sterilizing cycles are very fast; sterilization can be completed in 20-45 minutes in most cases. Delicate instruments and electrical equipment should not be steam autoclaved because of their sensitivity to water and heat and the potential for damage. Additionally, steam autoclaves can dull sharp cutting surfaces of scissors and other expensive medical instruments.

of peroxide to sterilize medical equipment. This technology is designed to be similar and less toxic than ethylene oxide; however, it is more expensive. Gamma radiation and electron beam sterilization are not widely utilized in veterinary medicine, although they have application in sterilization of healthcare products as well as food. Pulsed light sterilizers are being used in human hospitals enabling surface sterilization of whole rooms. Microwave and ozone gas can be used to sterilize equipment, but they provide limited penetrability.

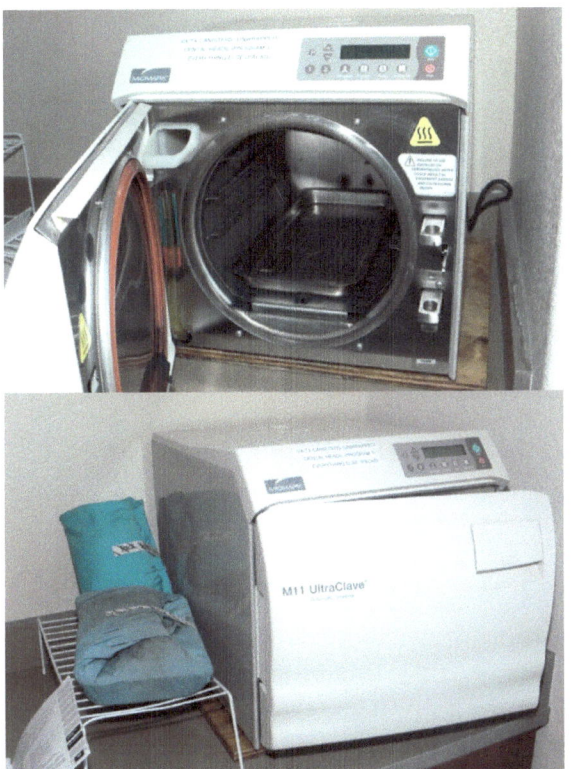

Figure 15: Steam autoclave interior and exterior

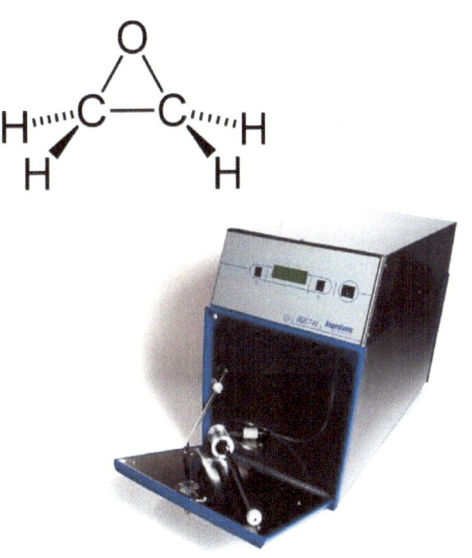

Figure 16: Ethylene oxide molecule and sterilizer

Ethylene oxide gas sterilization is useful for sterilizing instruments and equipment not suited for the steam autoclave. These items include delicate plastics and electronics, as well as fiber optic endoscopes. Ethylene oxide is a known carcinogen, so proper training and handling is imperative when utilizing this sterilization process. Peroxide sterilizers use the gas plasma-oxidative properties

Steam autoclaves can sterilize durable surgical instruments, drapes and gowns. Delicate instruments and equipment that can melt should not be sterilized in a steam autoclave.

Medical Terminology

Medical terminology is the vocabulary of medical conditions, anatomical features and medical processes of humans and animals. Medical terminology has an extensive history in the Greek and Latin languages and many of the words are derived from them. Specific terms are used to identify anatomical structures, diagnoses, instruments, procedures, protocols and medicines. The easiest way to decipher these words is by breaking them into parts. This is accomplished by recognizing the root word, prefix and suffix.

- The root word is usually derived from the source language and usually describes a body part.
- The prefix gives further information about the location, condition, or other specifics of the root word.
- The suffix can help further describe the condition, procedure, study, or disease process of the root word.

Once broken down, many difficult and unfamiliar medical terms can be more easily understood. Here are some examples.

Hypodermic needle
- Hypo (prefix)=below or under
- Dermic (root word)=referring to the dermis or skin

A hypodermic needle is used on a syringe to deliver medication under the skin.

Intramuscular injection
- Intra (prefix)=within
- Muscular (root word)=muscle

An intramuscular injection is a shot given into the muscle of the patient.

Bradycardia
- Brady (prefix)=slow
- Cardia (root word)=referring to the heart

Bradycardia refers to a slow heart rate.

Hyperglycemia
- Hyper (prefix)=increased or excessive
- Glyc (root word)=referring to sugar or glucose
- Emia (suffix)=referring to the blood

Hyperglycemia is a condition where an excessive amount of glucose is in the blood. Hyperglycemia is common in people and animals with diabetes.

Thrombocytopenia
- Thrombo (prefix)=referring to thrombus or clot
- Cyto (root word)=cell
- Penia (suffix)=referring to lack of or deficiency

Thrombocytopenia refers to a lack of clotting cells called thrombocytes (also known as platelets).

Ovariohysterectomy
- Ovario (prefix)=referring to the ovaries
- Hyster (root word)=pertaining to the uterus
- Ectomy (suffix)=surgical removal

Ovariohysterectomy is the surgical removal of the ovaries and uterus, and is commonly called a spay.

Prefix	Meaning	Example
a, an	without	asystole
abdo	abdomen	abdominal
anti	against, opposite	antibacterial
brady	slow	bradycardia
cardi	heart	cardiopulmonary
contra	against	contraception
cysto	bladder	cystocentisis
de	from, down, away	declaw
dys	difficult, troubled	dyspnea
gastro	stomach	gastrointestinal
hemo	blood	hemostasis
hyper	high, excessive	hyperthyroid
hypo	low, insufficient	hypodermic
intra	into	intravenous
osteo	bone	osteoporosis
poly	many	polyuria
pyo	pus	pyometra
tachy	fast	tachycardia

Suffix	Meaning	Example
centesis	to puncture, tap	cystocentesis
crit	separate	hematocrit
cyte	cell	leukocyte
ectomy	excise, Sx removal	splenectomy
emia	blood	anemia
esthesia	sensation	anesthesia
iasis	infestation	giardiasis
ism	condition, disease	hyperthyroidism
itis	inflammation	cellulitis
logy	study, practice	oncology
megaly	enlarged	cardiomegaly
oma	tumor	carcinoma
osis	abnormal condition	keratosis
pathy	disease	cardiopathy
penia	deficiency	cytopenia
phylaxis	protection	anaphylaxis
pnea	breath	dyspnea
pexy	surgical fixation	nephropexy
rrhea	flowing	diarrhea
rrhaphy	Sx repair, joining seam	tarsorrhaphy
stasis	stopping, constant	hemostasis
stenosis	narrowing	tracheal stenosis
stomy	make new opening	tracheostomy
tomy	incise, incision	laparotomy

Medical Terminology- General

ADR	Ain't doing right	**HCT**	Hematocrit
ASAP	As soon as possible	**Hx**	History
BAR	Bright, alert and responsive	**ICU**	Intensive care unit
BM	Bowel movement	**LRS**	Lactated ringers solution
BP	Blood pressure	**mm**	Mucous membrane
BW	Body weight	**MRI**	Magnetic resonance imaging
C&S	culture and sensitivity	**NPO**	No per os
Cast	Castration	**NSF**	No significant findings
CBC	Complete blood count	**OFA**	Orthopedic foundation of America
CNS	Central nervous system	**OTC**	Over the counter
COB	Care of body	**OVH/OHE**	Ovariohysterectomy
CPR	Cardiopulmonary resuscitation	**PCV**	Packed cell volume
CRT	Capillary refill time	**PDQ**	Pretty darn quick
CSF	Cerebral spinal fluid	**PU/PD**	Polyuria/polydypsia
DIC	Disseminated intravascular coagulation	**Px**	Prognosis
DJD	Degenerative joint disease	**qns**	Quantity not sufficient
DLH	Domestic long-hair	**R/O**	Rule out
DOA	Dead on arrival	**RACL**	Ruptured anterior cruciate ligament
DOB	Date of birth	**RAD**	Radiograph
DSH	Domestic short-hair	**RBC**	Red blood cell
DTM	Dermatophyte test medium	**RR**	Respiration rate
DVM	Doctor of Veterinary Medicine	**RV**	Rabies virus
Dx	Diagnosis	**RVT**	Registered Veterinary Technician
EAG	Express anal glands	**SOAP**	Subjective, objective, assessment, plan
ECG/EKG	Electrocardiogram	**sp.**	Species
EDTA	Ethylene diamine tetraacetic acid	**SR**	Suture removal
EENT	Eyes, ears, nose and throat	**STAT**	Statum
ER	Emergency room	**Sx**	Surgery
FB	Foreign body	**TP**	Total protein
FeLV	Feline leukemia virus	**TPR**	Temperature, pulse, respiration
FIP	Feline infectious peritonitis	**Tx**	Treatment
FIV	Feline immunodeficiency virus	**UA**	Urinalysis
FUO	Fever of unknown origin	**URI**	Upper respiratory infection
FUS	Feline urologic syndrome	**UTI**	Urinary tract infection
Fx	Fracture	**VA**	Veterinary assistant
GI	Gastro-intestinal	**V-D**	Ventro-dorsal
GDV	Gastric dilatation-volvulous	**WBC**	White blood cell
HBC	Hit by car	**WNL**	Within normal limits

Several useful medical terms for patient orientation are commonly used in veterinary medicine. These terms describe surfaces or regions of the body. This enables one to identify with specificity where, for example, a tumor is located on a pet. These terms are frequently used when describing animal positioning for radiographs.

Term	Refers to:
Cranial	Towards the front or head
Caudal	Towards the rear or tail
Dorsal	Towards the dorsum or back
Ventral	Towards the ventrum or belly
Proximal	Close to the body
Distal	Away from the body
Anterior	The front side of the limb
Posterior	The back side of the limb
Lateral	The surfaces of the sides
Medial	The surfaces on the insides

Table 2: Medical terms used to describe location on the body

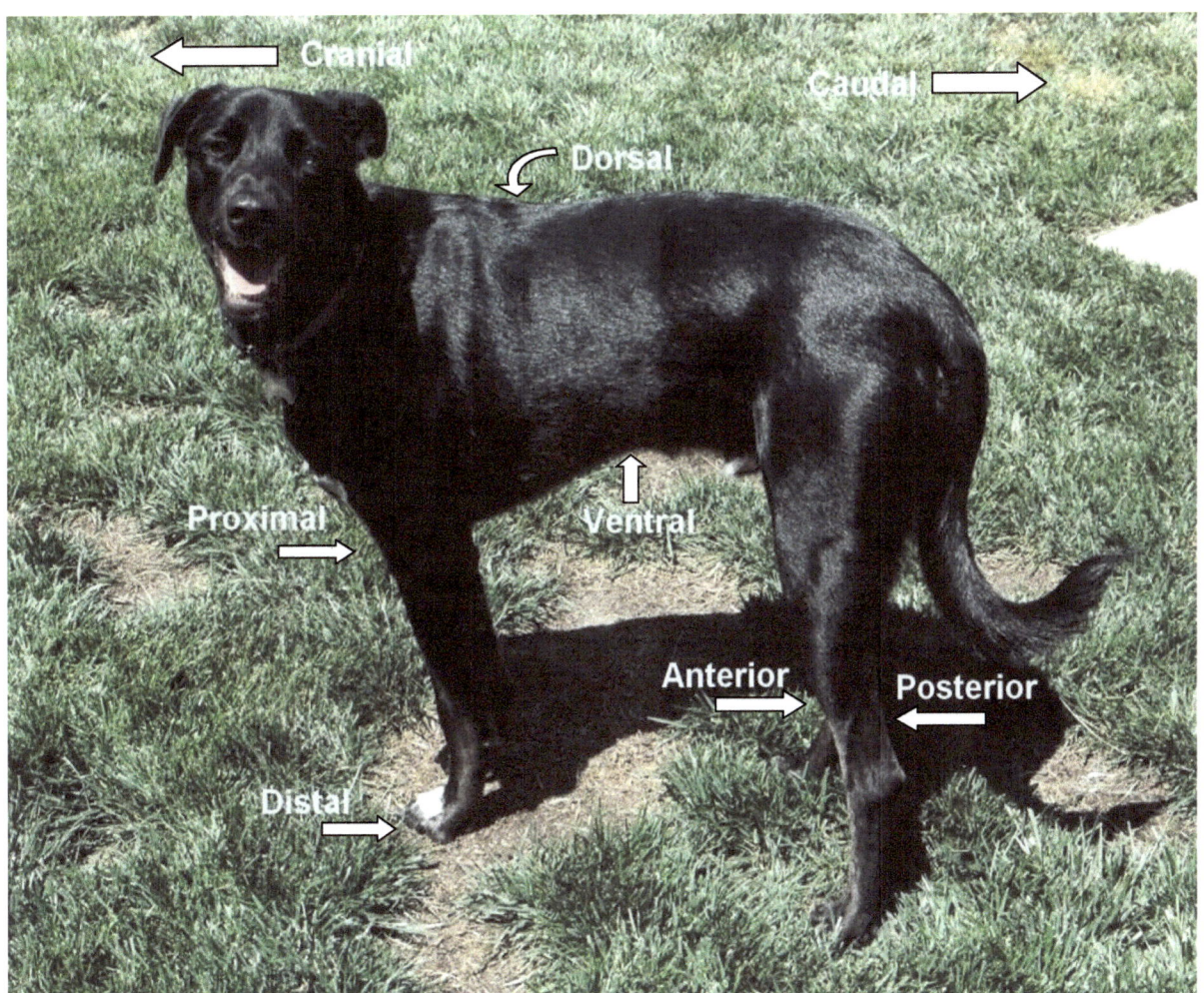

Figure 3: Terms used to describe patient orientation

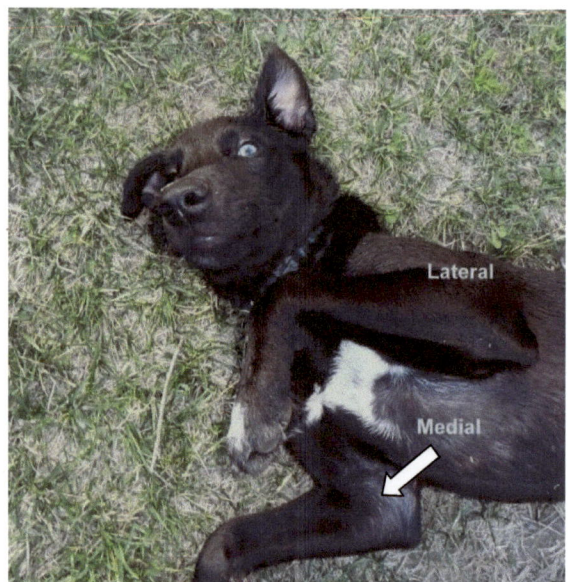
Figure 4: Terms used to describe the outside and inside surfaces of an animal

Many anatomical terms are used to describe parts of the body. Some of these terms are used interchangeably to describe a variety of anatomical structures.

Anatomical Term	Also Known As:
Chest	Thorax
Scruff	Interscapular
Knee	Stifle
Heel	Hock
Ear	Pinna

Table 5: Interchangeable anatomical terms

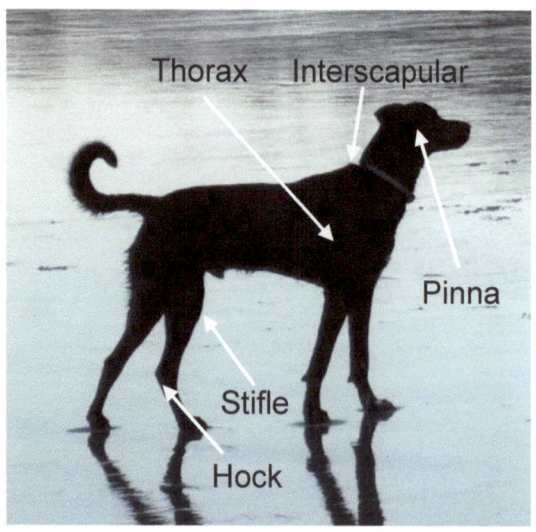

Acronyms and abbreviations are used in situations to convey information while using less writing. Many long words can be abbreviated in an attempt to save time when writing in a medical record or prescribing medication. Many abbreviations used in veterinary medicine are similar to those used in human medicine; although, some are quite unique to animal care. Here are a few you should know by now.

- DVM
- RVT
- VA

Special abbreviations are used when filling a prescription. Depending on the particular drug, some medications can be given several times daily; therefore, there are a variety of abbreviations used to identify medication frequency based on the doctor's prescription.

R$_x$	Prescription
PO	Per os or by mouth (orally)
SID	Once daily
BID	Twice daily
TID	Three times daily
QID	Four times daily
q	Every
EOD	Every other day
PRN	As needed

Table 6: Common abbreviations used for prescriptions

If a doctor wants to have a patient receive 1 tablet of a drug twice daily for 10 days, it could be abbreviated as:
1 tab PO BID x 10 days

If a doctor wants to have a patient receive 1 capsule of a drug every 3 days for 10 days, it could be abbreviated as:
1 cap PO q3d x 10 days

Other abbreviations relating to medications and prescriptions may include:

- Tab=tablet
- Cap=capsule
- Susp=suspension
- Oint=ointment
- Ophth=ophthalmic

Abbreviations are used to describe the eyes and ears. These terms can be used in prescriptions or as a means to communicate information relating to them in the medical record.

OD	Right eye (oculus dexter)
OS	Left eye (oculus sinister)
OU	Both eyes (oculus uterque)
AD	Right ear (auris dexter)
AS	Left ear (auris sinister)
AU	Both ears (auris uterque)

Table 7: Abbreviations for eyes and ears

Abbreviations for units of measure are used frequently in veterinary medicine. Units of measure are used in prescriptions and drug dosing, as well as anatomical measurements of structures such as tumors or lacerations. Worldwide, the metric system is preferred and more widely used; therefore, understanding both metric and US customary units is important. The metric system will be discussed in further detail in 'Medical Math'.

tsp	Teaspoon
tbs	Tablespoon
oz	Ounce
gal	Gallon
lb	Pound
cc	Cubic centimeter
ml	Milliliter
µl	Microliter
ℓ	Liter
µg	Microgram
mg	Milligram
g	Gram
kg	Kilogram
meq	Milliequivalents

Table 8: Abbreviations for common measures

Medical Records

The medical record documents a patient's medical history and care. Included in the medical record are notations about diagnoses and treatments, so that continuity of care can be maintained. Additionally, communication between veterinarian and owner can be documented, as well as any other information necessary for completeness. Remember, that because it is a legal document, the medical record should only be written in pen. Pencil or white-out should never be used; cross out incorrect entries with a single line through them. Furthermore, medical records and accompanying radiographs, must be kept by the clinic for at least three years. Each state has a version of the Veterinary Practice Act. This document characterizes the minimum requirements for a medical record. This includes:

- Name, address, phone number of animal's owner
- Name/identity of animal
- Age, sex, and breed of animal
- Dates of custody
- History of animal's condition
- Diagnosis of condition
- Medication and treatment, including amount and frequency
- Progress on disposition of case
- Surgical notations

Anatomy of a Medical Record
The client and pet information page, filled out by the pet's owner, provides personal information about the owner and pet. Pet information includes current medications, allergies and vaccine history. This information is filled out at the pet's first visit to the veterinary clinic.

Obtaining referral information is a valuable way for the clinic to determine marketing strategies and its effectiveness.

Blank medical record pages provide the ability to make medical entries about the patient. The entry starts with the day's date, followed by the reason for the pet's visit. Additional entries about the pet's condition can then be made. Entries regarding phone and other conversations can be recorded on this page. Additionally, entries regarding attitude, treatment, progress and health, can be made daily for hospitalized patients.

The master problem page summarizes patient vaccine and medical history. This enables the veterinarian to quickly see important medical conditions without having to scroll through the entire medical record.

Electronic medical records continue to be integrated into the veterinary workplace. These record systems provide flexibility, as well as ease of storage and sharing of medical information. Disadvantages include: startup costs, user learning curve and a lack of standardized terminology. Most electronic practice management software utilizes the same information on which paper based systems rely; this means that both of these record systems are functionally very similar.

Other Related Medical Forms
Several medical forms can be contained in a patient's medical record. Most diagnostic laboratory testing is reported on such a form, whether the testing is processed within the clinic or at an offsite facility. Common laboratory forms

may be generated from the following diagnostic tests:

- Complete blood count and biochemistry profiles
- Blood cultures
- Urinalysis
- Histology
- Cytology
- Tissue biopsies

Several other non-laboratory forms can be found in a medical record, they include:

- Rabies form
  - Used to verify rabies vaccination as a part of state licensing requirements
  - Fee discounted for altered pets
  - Currently only required for dogs
- Euthanasia form
  - Authorizes pet euthanasia by legal owner
  - Stipulates that no bites have occurred within 10 to 15 days
- Health certificate
  - Used for interstate and international wellness verification and rabies vaccination status
- Client estimate for services
  - Used to verify agreement of services to be provided by the veterinarian
  - Signed by pet owner, agreeing to pay for services
  - Prudent business practice, but not required

Figure 17: Generic rabies vaccination form

EUTHANASIA CONSENT FORM

Owner's Name: _____ Date: _____
Address: _____ Phone: _____
Street _____ Alt. Phone: _____
City _____ State/Zip_____
Pet's Name: _____ Breed: _____
Sex: _____ Age: _____ Color/Markings:_____

I, the undersigned, do hereby certify that I am the owner or duly authorized agent for the owner of the animal described above, that I do hereby give _____ (veterinarian) and his employees or representative, full and complete authority to end the life and dispose of said animal in whatever manner they shall deem appropriate.

I acknowledge that Dr. _____ has met with me personally and discussed the euthanasia of my animal. I also certify that to the best of my knowledge the said animal has not bitten any person or animal during the last fifteen (15) days, and has not been exposed to rabies. I further understand that I assume financial responsibility for all services rendered.

Again, by signing this form I am giving permission to end this animal's life and I have the authority to execute this consent.

_____ Date:_____
Signature of Owner or Agent

Figure 18: Generic euthanasia form

Anatomy and Physiology of Mammals

There are thirty-six animal phyla in the animal kingdom. Each phylum can be considered a group that shares the same overall body plan, which includes both external appearance and internal organization. Class mammalia is further grouped into those vertebrate animals that possess hair, three middle ear bones and mammary glands. There are over four-thousand extant species of mammals; dogs, cats and humans are in this class of mammals. The relationship between exotic and domesticated animals, as well as humans, makes understanding their anatomy and physiology easier. By learning the anatomy and physiology of a dog or cat, you are ultimately learning the workings of exotics as well as yourself.

Dogs (canids) and cats (felids) possess more similarities in structure and function than differences. They also possess similarities to humans; differences include their tails and quadruped locomotion. Anatomy is the study of these internal and external structures and physiology is the study of how they work. Here are some valuable animal structures starting from the cellular level.

Cells are the fundamental component of all tissues and organs. Cells possess a nucleus containing DNA (deoxyribonucleic acid). DNA contains the genetic material necessary for cellular replication and function. These processes require both food and oxygen to the cells. Digested food provides the nutrients and respiration provides the oxygen.

Cell types include:
- Epithelial cells
    - These cells make up skin and line cavities and surfaces of structures in the body.
- Connective cells
    - These cells include bone, cartilage and blood.
- Muscle cells
    - These cells are considered smooth, skeletal, or cardiac and are used to contract muscles, the heart, or intestines.
- Nervous cells
    - These cells conduct electrical signals.

Blood cells are important to understand as they are a valuable diagnostic source of animal wellness. Variations in cell types or proportions can be indicative of disease or illness. These connective tissue cells include:
- Red blood cells or RBC's
- White blood cells or WBC's
- Platelets or thrombocytes

Together, these cells make up about thirty-five to forty-five percent of the blood tissue volume. This percentage of cell volume is called the hematocrit or packed cell volume (PCV). The white blood cell portion is sometimes referred to as the buffy coat, and the non-cellular portion is called serum.

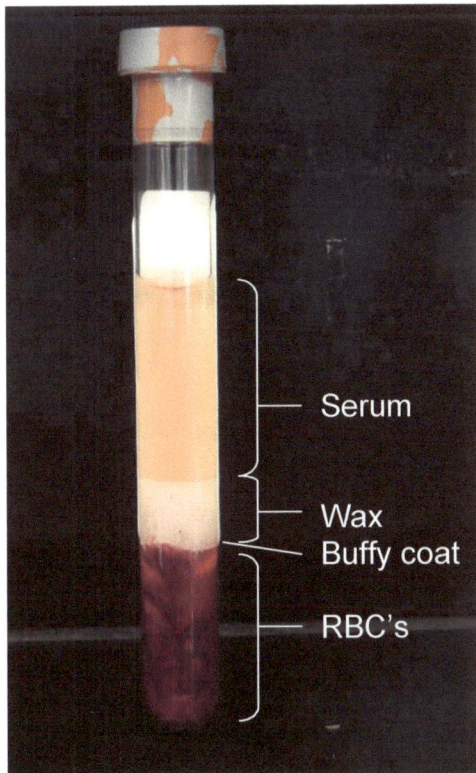

Figure 19: Blood tube showing the RBC's separated from the serum by a piece of wax

Red blood cells or erythrocytes, function to provide oxygen to the tissues of the body. They also serve to remove some carbon dioxide from the body. They are produced in the bone marrow and some are stored in the spleen. They have a lifespan of about 120 days and lack a nucleus at maturity. RBC's are the most numerous of all the blood cells and make up nearly ninety-nine percent of the PCV. RBC's are about six to eight microns in diameter (0.0003 inches).

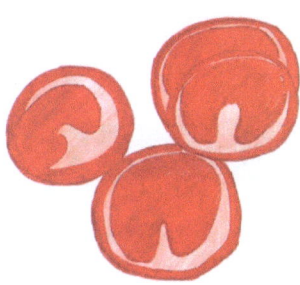

Figure 20: Red blood cells

White blood cells or leukocytes are cells of the immune system and function to fight infection and foreign material. The number of WBC's in the blood is often an indicator of disease. WBC's are composed of five cell types:

- Neutrophil
    - Two to three times the size of a RBC
    - Defends against bacterial or fungal infections
    - Major component of pus
    - Makes up 60-70% of all WBC's

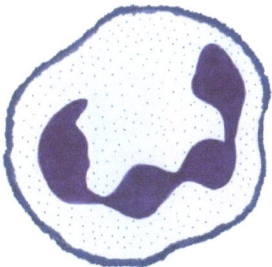

- Lymphocyte
    - Slightly larger than a RBC
    - 3 types make antibodies, help kill pathogens, cancer cells and virus infected cells

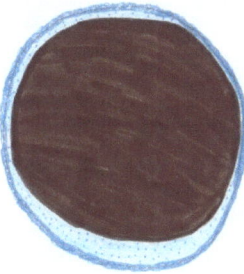

- Monocyte
    - Two to three times the size of a RBC
    - Eats cells by process called phagocytosis
    - Long lived leukocyte

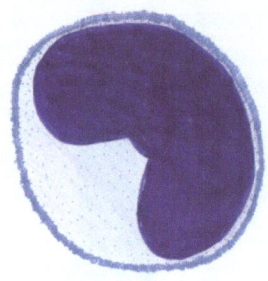

- Eosinophil
  - Two to three times the size of a RBC
  - Responds to parasitic infections and allergic reactions

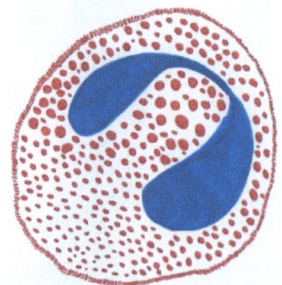

- Basophil
  - Two to three times the size of a RBC
  - Involved in allergic and antigen response

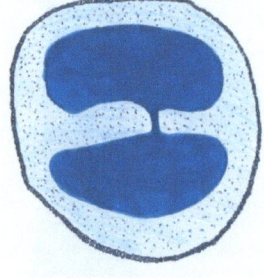

Platelets or thrombocytes are responsible for blood clotting. They create a mesh that red blood cells stick to in order to stop more blood from leaving the body. Reductions in platelets can lead to bleeding disorders like hemophilia. Some toxins affect the body's ability to clot. A single platelet is about one third the size of a RBC.

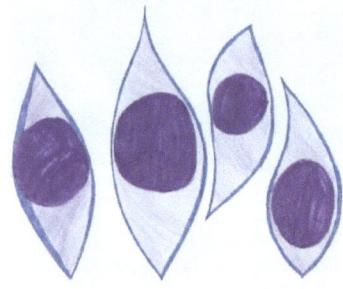

Figure 21: Platelets

Over fifty percent of whole blood is non-cellular. This fluid matrix is made up of mostly water, but also contains nutrients, proteins and waste products such as carbon dioxide and urea. Blood plasma also carries electrolytes such as sodium and chloride, albumin, oxygen, immunoglobulins and clotting factors. Changes in blood plasma can be seen in the PCV; a higher PCV can be indicative of dehydration.

The Skeletal System of Dogs and Cats

The vertebrate skeleton provides support; is designed as scaffolding for muscles and affords protection for internal organs of the body. Bone is the rigid connective tissue that makes up the skeleton. Some bone produces blood cells and acts as a source of minerals necessary for the body. Cartilage, an inflexible connective tissue similar to bone, is also found in many areas of the body. The numbers of bones in the body differ by species, but the functions of the bones are often times considered homologous. For example, the leg of a human is homologous to the leg of a dog.

The adult human skeleton contains 206 bones. The dog and cat have about 320 bones; the tail making up the difference in numbers. The skeletal system can be separated into two categories, those of the axial and appendicular skeleton.

Bones of the axial skeleton or midline include the skull, vertebrae, ribs and tail. The appendicular skeleton includes the bones of the shoulders, arms, pelvis and legs. They are also known as the appendages or limbs.

Skeletal connections of bones enable movement of the body; muscles contract against bones causing motion. Some bones connect to joints. Types of joints include those that pivot, hinge, or are a ball and socket. Ligaments are tough fibrous connective tissues that help hold these joints together with stability. Ligaments, therefore, connect bones together; synovial fluid and cartilaginous pads prevent bones and joints from grinding together. Tendons are similar to ligaments; however, they connect muscle bundles to bone.

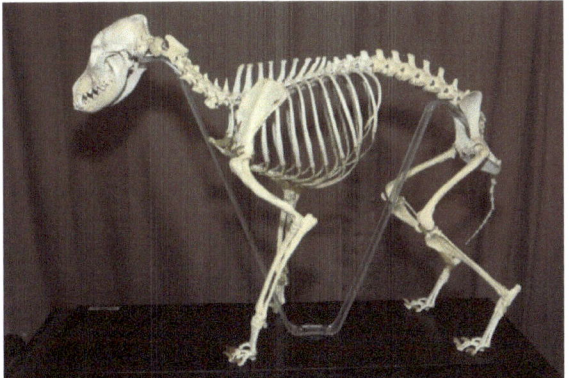

Figure 22: Dog skeleton

Learning all the names of the bones in dogs, means you are learning the names of all the bones in you....except the tail!

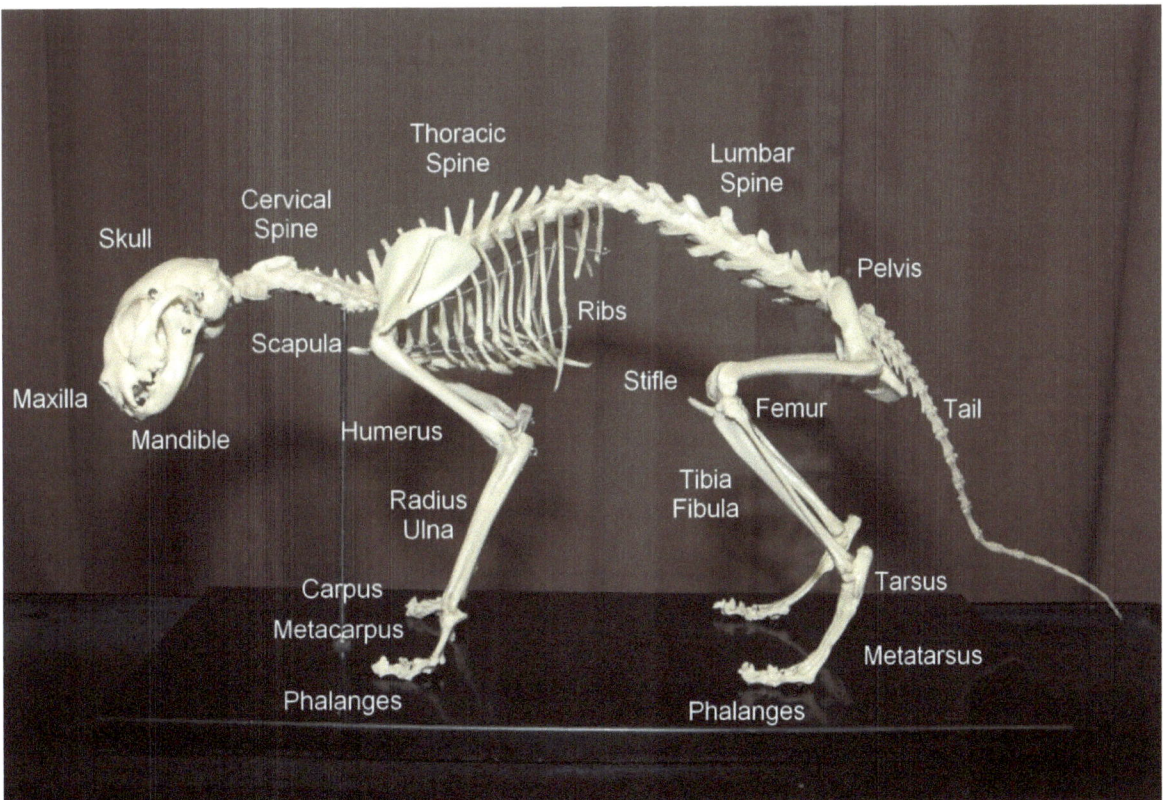

Figure 23: Names of the bones of the cat

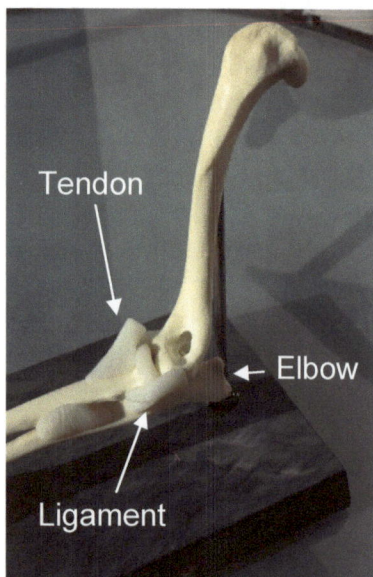

Figure 24: Elbow joint showing ligament connecting bone to bone and tendon connecting bone to muscle (bicep muscle not shown)

The integumentary system is a sensory system that regulates temperature by use of piloerection of hair and production of sweat. Skin, hair, nails, feathers and scales make up the integumentary system. Skin is considered the largest organ and provides protection, detects pain, temperature and pressure, as well as provides weatherproofing. Skin is composed of three layers, they include:

- Epidermis
- Dermis
- Subdermis or subcutaneous layer

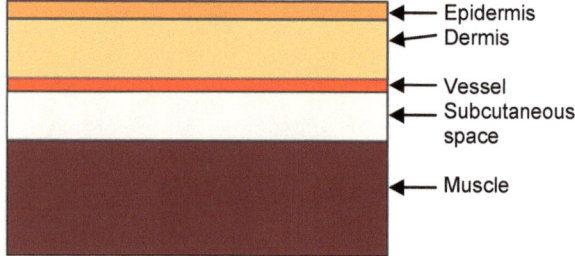

Figure 25: Skin layers

Hair, grown from follicles in the dermis, is made up of keratinized cells that protect skin from the environment, provide insulation and have sensory

properties. Hair can also make an animal look larger, making it a means of defense. Claws, hoofs, horns, quills and beaks are all specialized hair made of keratin.

The *nervous system* is composed of the brain, spinal cord, nerves and nerve endings. The primary role of the nervous system is to communicate information to cells via nerve conduction and transmission.

The *circulatory system* is an organ system which provides the body's cells with nutrients, gases and hormones through a series of pipes throughout the body. Blood is the transport fluid; the heart is the pump. The circulatory system can also be viewed as a busy freeway system where the cars are the blood cells, and as the cars get off the freeway they go down smaller roads and side streets until they get to their destination. If functioning properly, the circulatory system will provide oxygen and nutrients to the organs and tissues of the body. Two easy ways of determining how well the tissues are being oxygenated can be found in the mucous membranes of the mouth. Mucous membrane (MM) color should be pink and not pale, if tissue perfusion is adequate. Additionally, capillary refill time (CRT) should take only a couple of seconds. CRT is determined by pressing on the mucous membranes, then lifting up your finger and counting the time in which the capillary beds refill with blood.

Arteries and Veins

Blood leaves the heart through an artery. Because the heart is pumping the blood with great force, the artery has very thick walls to prevent rupture from the pressure. Blood continues through the artery until it reaches the tissue capillaries; oxygen and nutrients are exchanged here. As the blood leaves the tissue, it is now oxygen and nutrient deprived. The blood leaves these tissues in veins; these are thin-walled vessels because there is less pressure as the blood returns to the heart. Arteries, veins and nerves will often times be near each other; arteries are usually deep under the muscles, and veins are usually near the skins surface.

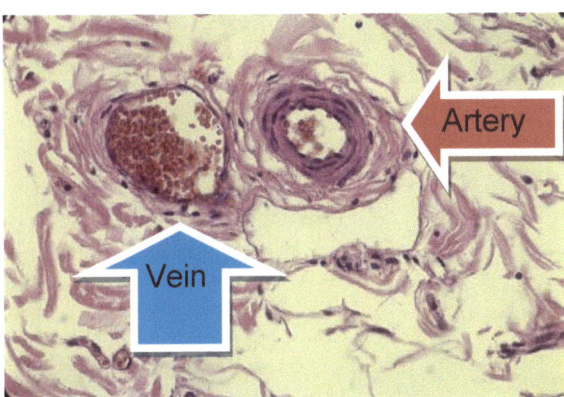

Figure 26: Artery and vein in cross section. Notice the difference in wall thickness.

Three important veins used in veterinary medicine include the cephalic, jugular, and saphenous veins.

The Heart

The mammalian heart is responsible for pumping blood throughout the vessels of the body. Blood is also pumped to the lungs so gas exchange can occur. The heart, in its simplest terms, can be viewed as two pumps; one pumping blood to the body, and the other pumping blood to the lungs. The mammalian heart has 4 chambers to perform this task. Two chambers prepare blood for pumping, and two do the actual pumping. Muscular

contractions of the heart, pump blood as a result of electrical impulses stimulating the heart to contract. An electrocardiogram or ECG graphically shows the electrical activity of the heart during contraction and relaxation. The ECG is useful in determining how well the heart is conducting electricity as well as how well blood is being pumped to the body.

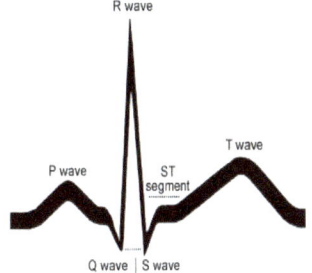

Figure 27: ECG tracing showing a single heart cycle. The QRS complex is a result of ventricular contraction.

The chambers on the top of the heart are called atria (singular=atrium), and the larger chambers below are called ventricles. Atria have thin walls and ventricles have thick walls. The left ventricle has thicker walls than the right. Valves separate the atria from the ventricles.

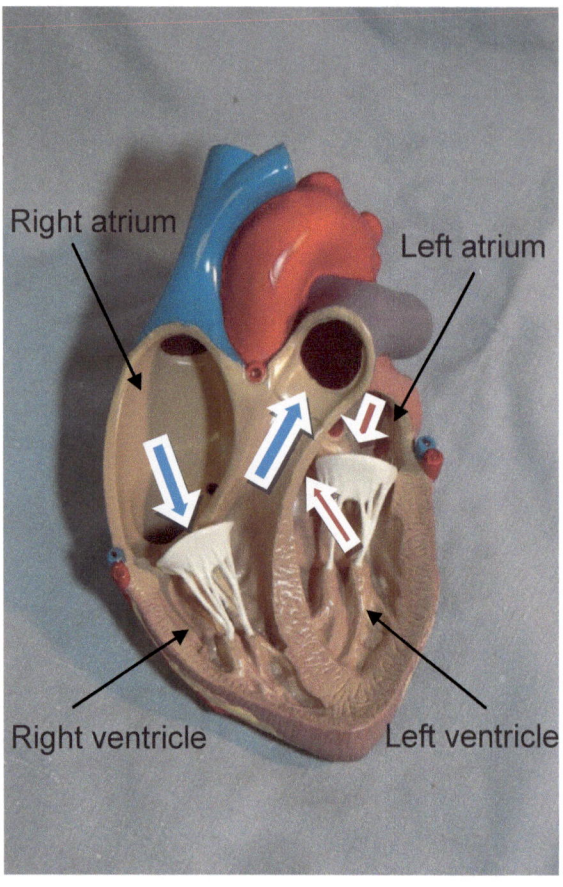

Right atrium

Left atrium

Right ventricle

Left ventricle

The Pathway Made Easy

Blood circulates through the body in less than thirty seconds. Here is how blood gets around.

1. Blood enters right atrium from the body
2. Blood is pumped to right ventricle
3. Blood is pumped to lungs
4. Oxygenation of blood occurs in the lungs
5. Blood returns to left atrium
6. Blood is pumped to left ventricle
7. Blood is pumped to the body

Specifically, both atria contract together; this is followed by contraction of both ventricles. This means that blood is entering both ventricles during atrial contraction, and blood is going to both the lungs and to the body during ventricular contraction.

Heart Sounds

The heartbeat can usually be felt by placing one's hand on the left side of the chest. The use of a stethoscope on the left side of an animal can make the task of hearing the heart even easier. The heart actually makes several sounds, two of which are very audible. These two sounds, a lub, followed by a dub, are usually heard. Each lub-dub constitutes one heart cycle, and is considered a single heartbeat. These two prominent sounds are a result of the closing of the heart valves. The first sound occurs after atrial contraction. As the atria relax, the valves between the atria and ventricles close. The second sound occurs after ventricular contraction. As the ventricle relax, the valves leaving the heart close. In summary:

- The first heart sound, or lub, occurs as a result of the closing of the valves between the atria and ventricles. These are known as the tricuspid and mitral valves.
- The second heart sound, or dub, occurs as a result of the closing of the valves that leave the heart. These are known as the aortic and pulmonic valves (semilunar).

Normal heart rates (HR) vary by species, but in general, smaller animals have faster heart rates, and larger animals have slower rates. Heart rates are always calculated as beats per minute. Remember, each lub-dub counts as one heartbeat, and counting the beats in one minute will determine the heart rate. To save time, count the beats in fifteen seconds and multiply that number by four; that will determine the heart rate in beats per minute. Abnormal heart sounds can occur and are noteworthy. These can be heard as a result of heart disease, drugs, or congenital defects of the heart. Heart murmurs can be present due to some drugs or as a result of heart valve defects. A murmur can sound like a swishing noise instead of a lub or dub. Additionally, abnormal heart rates should be documented. Bradycardia is defined as a slow heart rate, and tachycardia, is a rapid heart rate.

> **The lub-dub heard when listening to the heart is a result of valves closing, and constitutes one heartbeat.**

Blood Pressure

The circulatory system is a closed system; blood leaves the heart via pipes and returns to the heart via pipes. As the heart contracts, an increase in blood pressure occurs. Upon relaxation of the heart, blood pressure drops. Systolic blood pressure refers to the pipe pressure during heart contraction. Diastolic, or resting blood pressure, refers to the pipe pressure during heart relaxation. Interestingly, most species, including humans, have similar blood pressure values. A normal blood pressure value is expressed as systolic pressure (SP) over diastolic pressure (DP). It is often written as SP/DP. A normal value is 120/70. A systolic pressure above 180 is considered hypertensive, and a diastolic pressure below 60 is considered hypotensive. An average blood pressure can be calculated based on the systolic and diastolic pressures. This average or mean arterial pressure (MAP) is often used as a convenient way of tracking blood pressure during anesthetic

procedures. The math can be calculated using the following equation:

- $MAP = 2/3DP + 1/3SP$

Blood pressure can be determined by two methods, these include invasive and non-invasive techniques.

- NIBP-non-invasive blood pressure utilizes a blood pressure cuff that is placed around a limb. The cuff is filled with air, and blood pressure is determined by occluding an artery. Once the artery is occluded, air is slowly released from the cuff until a pulse is heard; that pressure is the SP. Air is allowed to continue to be released until the pulse is no longer heard; that pressure is the DP.
- IBP-invasive blood pressure utilizes a catheter placed directly into an artery. This is a precise measurement of blood pressure.

In both cases, special equipment is used to determine the numerical blood pressure values. NIBP systems are convenient to attach and utilize, and therefore are most commonly seen in veterinary practices. Although, not as accurate as IBP monitoring, NIBP values are comparable. Thick hair coats and hypothermia can make NIBP values more difficult to obtain.

Pulse Rate

The pressure generated by the dub of ventricular heart contraction causes a pulse or surge in arterial pressure in other areas. A pulse can be felt at many locations on the body. Blood pressure monitoring systems use the pulse to determine both systolic and diastolic pressure. Several locations can be used to determine pulse rate and quality in animals:

- Femoral pulse can be felt on the inside of the back limbs near the pelvis
- Pedal pulse can be felt on the inside of the rear digits
- Axillary pulse can be felt on the inside of the front limbs near the chest

> **The heart rate and pulse rate should be the same value; remember, each lub-dub constitutes 1 heartbeat.**

Respiration

The *respiratory system* of mammals begins at the nose, and ends at the lungs. The function of the respiratory system is to provide gas exchange between the outside environment and the circulatory system. This exchange includes the acquisition of oxygen (O_2) for the body, and removal of carbon dioxide gas (CO_2) from the body. Respiration also allows for animals to vocalize; thus, communicate with each other.

The nose is the location of olfaction or the sense of smell. Additionally, the nose functions to condition air entering and leaving the body. This means that cold air entering the body can be warmed, and humidity can be preserved from air leaving the body. This is done by the use of turbinates; these skin folds significantly increase the surface area in the nose. Inspired air enters the nose and proceeds to the back of the throat or pharynx. Here, it reaches the entrance of the trachea. The trachea is a cartilaginous ringed tube that enables air to travel to the lungs. Cartilaginous rings ensure that the trachea does not collapse and prevent the flow of air. The entrance of the trachea has a structure called the epiglottis. The epiglottis functions to cover the trachea between respirations. It also closes over the trachea during food intake; this ensures that no food enters the lungs. The trachea terminates at the carina. This bifurcation splits the trachea off into the two bronchi of the lungs. Lungs are the location of O_2 exchange. Alveoli in the lungs enable blood (RBC's) to come in close contact with O_2. Carbon dioxide, a toxic gas produced by cell metabolism, is exchanged for oxygen by the RBC's. CO_2 is then removed by exhalation. The net result is as follows:

- O_2 is brought in by inspiration
- O_2 is bound by red blood cells at the alveoli
- CO_2 is removed by expiration

The diaphragm, a thin muscle separating the chest from the abdomen, facilitates respiration. Contraction of the diaphragm pulls the lungs in a negative pressure environment and causes inspiration or lung filling. Relaxation of the diaphragm allows for the expiration of air. The respiration rate (RR) of the animal is determined by the number of times respiration occurs in one minute, and is commonly denoted as breaths per minute. In general, the larger the animal the slower the respiration rate.

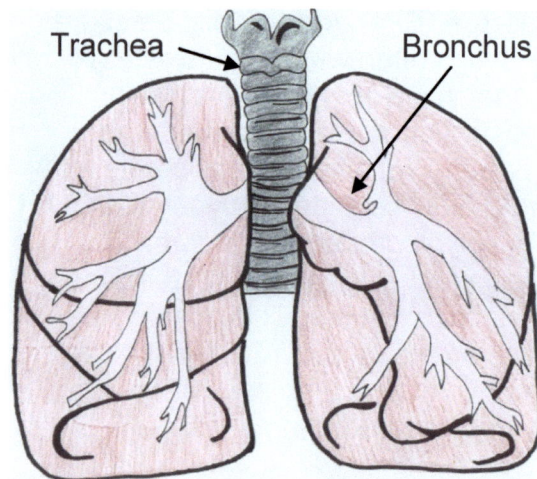

Figure 28: Lungs, bronchi, and trachea

O_2 and CO_2 have significant effects on the respiratory system and the body. An increase in CO_2 stimulates respiration as the body attempts to remove this toxic gas. High levels of CO_2 can eventually cause respiratory arrest and death. Normal environmental O_2 levels at sea level are about twenty percent; the body uses about thirteen percent of that. O_2 levels, however, decrease at higher elevations. High levels of O_2 can cause apnea because of a lack of CO_2 stimulation. Medical grade oxygen, used for anesthetic procedures, contains one hundred percent O_2.

Digestion

The *digestive system* is a mechanical and chemical process where food is broken down into usable components by the body. Digestion begins at the mouth. Here, food is chewed by teeth, and begins to be chemically broken down by saliva. The material then travels down the esophagus to the stomach. The esophagus is a flexible tube that can accommodate varying sizes of food. The stomach is the site of primary digestion. The acidic environment allows for the further breakdown of the food; hydrochloric acid is responsible for this process. In dogs and cats, this process may take four to six hours.
Bile, produced by the liver and stored in the gall bladder, aids in digestion of food in the small intestine. The small intestine is responsible for absorption of most of the nutrients produced by digestion. The large intestine removes water from the remaining digesta and stores the remaining material as feces. The rectum is the location of this storage area; elimination occurs when feces passes through the anus.

Excretion

The *excretory system* functions to remove toxins, water and unnecessary nutrients from the body in the form of urea (urine). Kidneys, bean shaped paired organs found in the dorsal abdomen, filter blood and remove wastes via the nephrons. These wastes, called urine, leave the kidneys and travel down the ureters to the bladder. Ureters essentially connect the kidneys to the bladder. The bladder stores urine produced by the kidneys until it is eliminated. The urethra is the drainage pipe for the bladder; it terminates at the penis or vulva and allows the bladder to be emptied.

Temperature is an important element of mammalian physiology. Endothermy, the process by which mammals maintain a consistent internal temperature, requires some form of energy. When an animal is cold, peripheral vessels close, and shivering may occur as a means to generate heat. In hot weather, animals may pant or sweat in an attempt to evaporate heat. Overall, however, a moderate temperature is maintained. Dogs and cats maintain a normal temperature range, running slightly warmer than humans. Temperatures between 100 and 102.5 can be considered normal. Temperatures above or below this range may be normal, but further investigation of activity or stress prior to temperature determination should be considered.

Eyes and Ears

The general anatomy of the dog and cat eye is similar to human's eye, however, there are some noteworthy differences. The eye contains an opening for light called the pupil; in cats, the pupil is more of a vertical slit than a round hole. The iris surrounds the pupil, dilating it in low light, and contracting it in bright light. The iris is usually brown, but may be blue or green in some species. The sclera is the white portion of the eye behind the iris. Dogs and cats have a structure in the back of the eye called the tapetum lucidum. This reflective structure causes their eyes to shine in the dark, and aids in low light vision. The eyes are protected by the upper and lower lids, as well as a nictitating membrane usually referred to as the third eyelid. The conjunctiva is the tissue surrounding the eye just under the protective upper and lower lids.

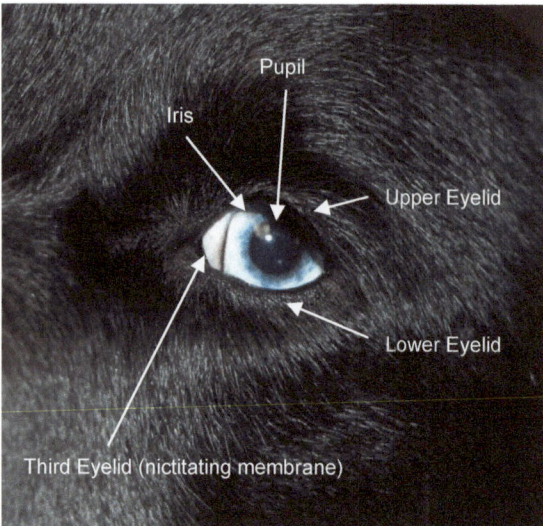

Figure 29: Anatomy of the dog eye

Dogs and cats have rods on the back surface of the eye or retina. Rods are photoreceptor cells sensitive to light and are especially important for nocturnal species. Cones, the second type of cells, are used for color vision. Dogs and cats have a limited number of cones (blue and green sensitive cones) suggesting that they have limited color vision.

The internal structures of the ear are synonymous in mammals, including dogs, cats and humans. The eardrum, a semitransparent membrane deep in the

auditory canal, can be visualized with a light emitting otoscope. The otoscope enables veterinarians the ability to determine if the eardrum is absent or has been damaged. Unlike humans, the auditory canal in dogs and cats turns upward, making visualization of the eardrum more challenging. Debris and foreign bodies such as foxtails can be seen with an otoscope. Foxtails can be a serious problem for pets in rural area or those that frequent areas where these plants grow. Head shaking and scratching at the ears may be indicative of an ear infection of foreign body.

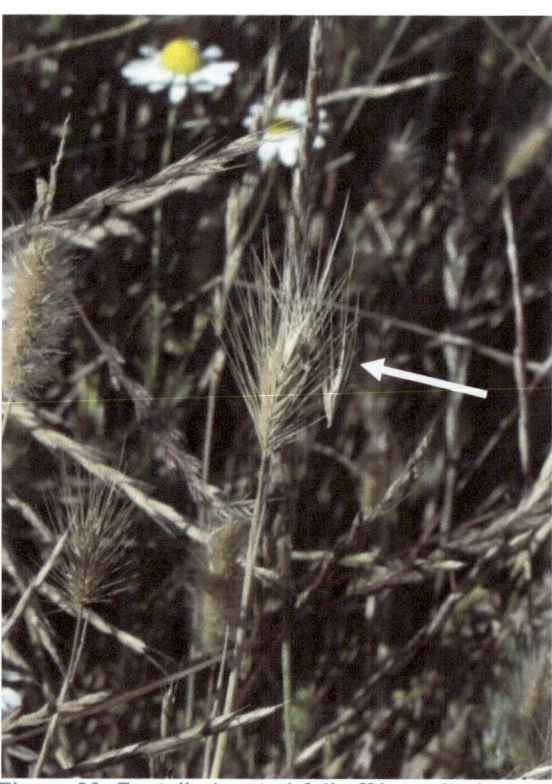

Figure 30: Foxtails (center) fall off into single small plantons.

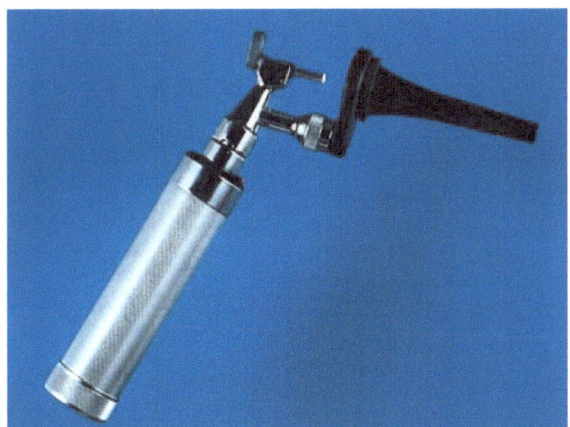
Figure 31: Otoscope with conical earpiece

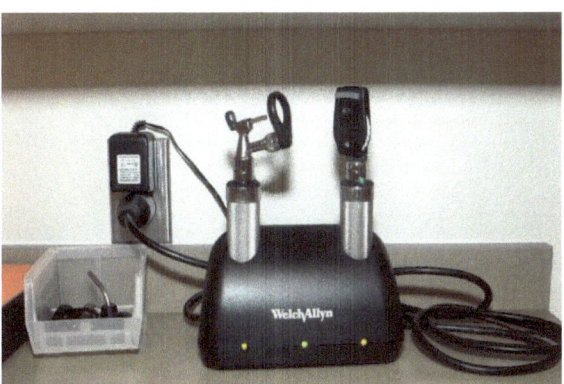
Figure 32: Otoscope (left) and ophthalmoscope

The external portion of the ear is called the pinna; it is variable in size and orientation depending on the species. Dogs with long floppy pinnas may experience more ear infections due to decreased airflow in the canal. Some breeds may also have hair in the auditory canal which may lead to chronic infection for the same reason. An aural hematoma, a blood filled pocket formed in the pinna from a ruptured blood vessel, is more commonly seen in dogs, and may require surgery to resolve.

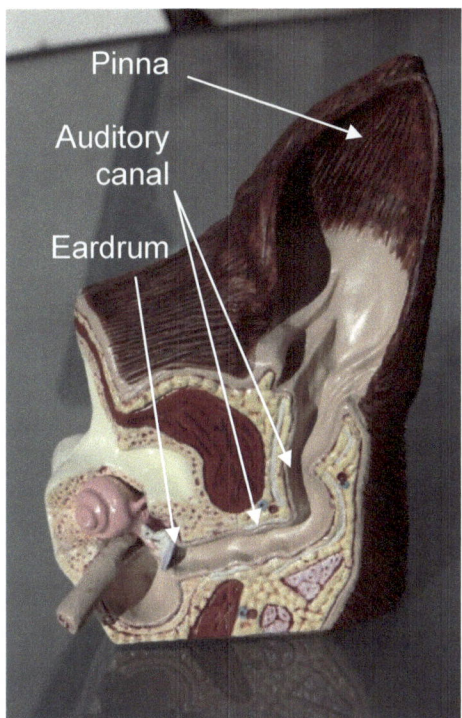
Figure 33: Structural anatomy of the dog and cat ear. Notice horizontal and vertical canal

Reproductive Anatomy

The reproductive anatomy of dogs and cats varies slightly, and requires understanding when determining neonatal gender or determining rectal temperatures. Common to both genders is the anus. The anus is the terminal end of the digestive system and is located just under the base of the tail. Anal glands, present on both sides of the anus, function to scent feces as it is being pushed out the anal sphincter. The anus is the site for rectal thermometer placement and temperature determination.

Female
Below (ventral to) the anus in the female dog and cat resides the external genitalia; the vulva is the termination of the vagina. The vulva may be red and swollen during estrus, and may have a heart-shaped appearance. Unlike the anus, the vagina is a clean environment, so care must be taken not to place a

rectal thermometer here. The bulk of the female reproductive anatomy resides in the abdomen; this includes the body of the uterus, ovaries and uterine horns. Because dogs and cats have large litters of offspring, the uterine horns are quite elongated, and are the location of fetal implantation.

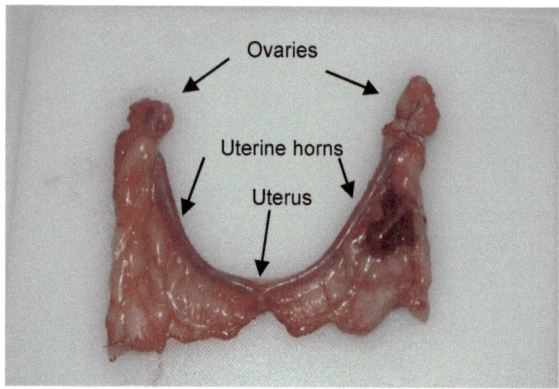

Figure 34: Uterus of the dog

Male

Below (ventral to) the anus in the male dog and cat resides the scrotum. The scrotum contains paired testicles which are the source of sperm for reproduction. A neuter involves the removal of the testicles, leaving the scrotum intact. Testicles in the neonate can be very small, but should be palpable during a physical exam. Cryptorchidism is described as the absence of one of the testicles in the scrotum; anorchidism is the lack of both testicles. Just below the scrotum in cats is the penis. The penis is very small in cats, and is oriented in a downward and caudal position. The penis can be extruded by putting pressure on either side of it, causing it to protrude. The penis in the dog is located on the ventral aspect of the abdomen. The base of the penis terminates at the scrotum. The penis is covered with a skin-covered sheath called a prepuce. Retraction of the prepuce towards the scrotum exposes the penis.

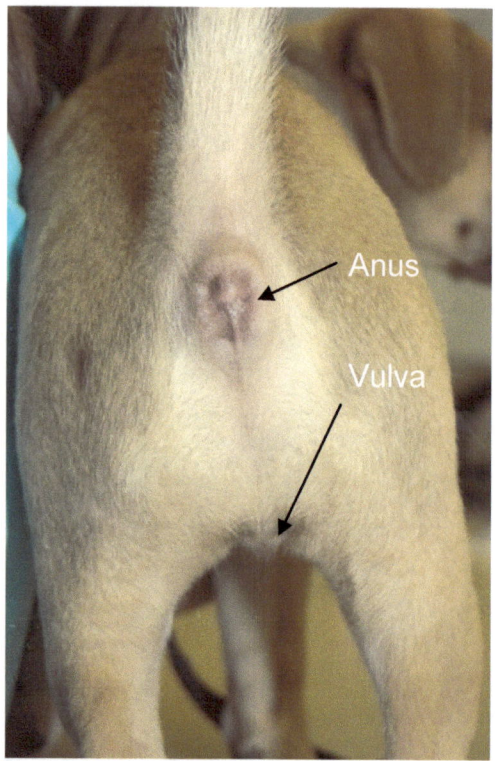

Figure 35: Female dog

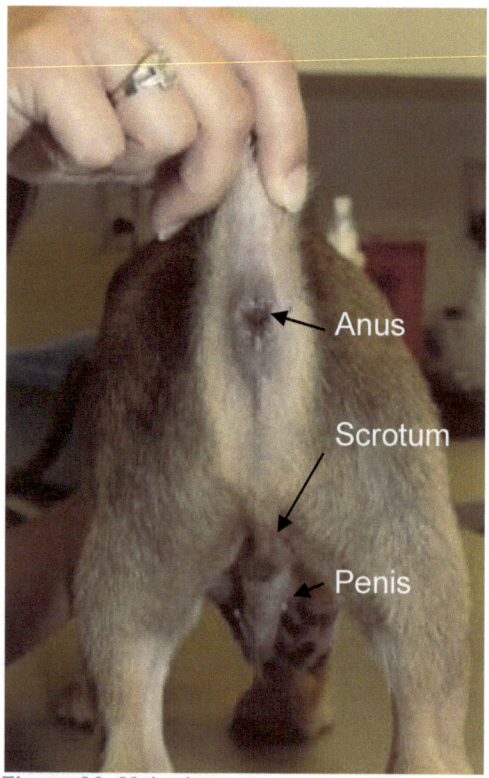

Figure 36: Male dog

Summary of the Organ Systems

Organ system	Organ	Function
Skeletal system	Bone	Gives body structure and ability to move. Marrow inside bones is responsible for red and white blood cell production.
Integumentary system	Skin	Provides a protective barrier for the bones and internal organs.
Circulatory system	Heart	Pumps blood to the body via arteries; blood returns to the heart through veins.
Respiratory system	Lungs	Exchange oxygen from the environment with carbon dioxide from the body.
Digestive system	Stomach	Food digestion using acidic bile (HCL) produced by the liver and stored in the gall bladder.
	Liver	Produces bile and processes nutrients and hormones to synthesize products used by the body.
	Pancreas	Regulates glucose in the body by producing insulin and glucagon. Aids in digestion of food.
	Small intestine	Primary area of nutrient absorption.
	Large intestine	Primary area of water re-absorption.
	Colon	Area where feces, the leftovers of digestion, are stored prior to defecation.
Excretory system	Kidneys	Paired organs responsible for the excretion of toxins and byproducts of digestion and metabolism in the blood. Excreted fluid called urine.
	Bladder	Urine produced by the kidneys leaves via the ureters and is stored in the bladder until it is eliminated from the body.
Nervous system	Brain	Central processing area for the body. The brain controls other organs by activating muscles or releasing hormones or neurotransmitters.
	Spinal cord	Enables sensory signals to be communicated back and forth between the brain and the body.
Lymphatic system	Spleen	Removes old red blood cells as well as RBC storage. It is also involved with the immune system and cleaning the blood of bacteria.

Physical Exam

The physical exam is a common procedure in veterinary medicine. The evaluation of animal wellness is important on a routine basis or when disease is present. The physical exam is a culmination of both historical and background information, as well as current status and physical evaluation. A pre-physical evaluation can be assessed prior to handling of the pet, and may include:

- The purpose for the visit
- The chief complaint or problem
- Vaccination history
- Current diet and changes in appetite
- Current medications
- Determination of breed
- Evaluation of appearance, coat, gait, mentation
- Determination of weight, size
- Determination of respiration rate

The physical exam involves evaluation of the patient's physical status and vital signs to establish an assessment of its condition. The veterinarian, with years of schooling and experience, is able to take historical information, behavior patterns and physical parameters to determine patient wellness. The veterinarian, usually, has a system of physical exam steps, taken so that no area is missed or under-evaluated. Because a veterinarian does so many exams, consistency in the exam process is very important. Many veterinarians begin their exam at the head of the patient. This satisfies the requirement of consistency, but also enables the veterinarian to properly greet the patient prior to physical manipulation. Here are some steps to consider, as well as areas to look at when doing a complete physical exam on a pet.

- Start cranial (front) to caudal (back)
- Greet patient, establish relationship
- Evaluate eyes, ears, nose, throat (EENT)
- Determine CRT, MM, tartar and dentition status
- Check skin for alopecia, psoriasis, masses, lesions
- Determine hydration
- Determine heart rate and quality, respiration rate and quality
- Check limbs for dissymmetry
- Check umbilicus for herniations
- Check for normal external genitalia
- Determine gender
- Determine temperature
- Check tail and perianal region

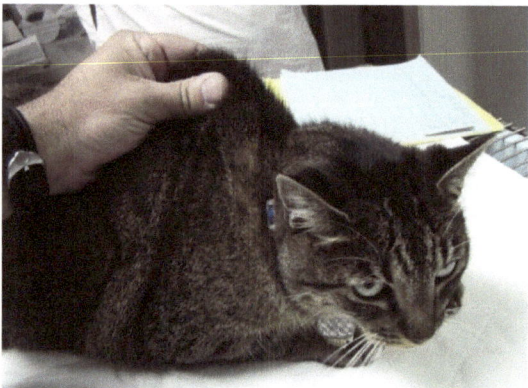

Figure 37: Hydration determination. Skin should spring back after release if hydration is normal.

	Temp (°F)	HR Beats/min	RR Breaths/min	MM	CRT (sec)
DOG	100-102.5	60-120	14-25	Pink	2
CAT	100-102.5	110-140	20-30	Pink	2

Table 9: Normal Dog and Cat Vital Signs

Handling and Restraint of Animals

Animal handling and restraint is the most important concept for veterinary support staff. This requires an understanding of animal behavior, knowledge of proper animal positioning, anatomical regions and locations, as well as effective use of restraint techniques and devices. Indications for restraint include patient control for procedures or examination. These procedures may be unpleasant or could cause harm to the animal; they may include blood or urine collection, medication administration, or wound care.

Procedures that may cause harm to the handler include those involving fearful or aggressive animals. Painful procedures may also elicit aggressive responses uncharacteristic of many animals. Recognizing certain behavior types enables the animal handler to predict how an animal might behave in any given situation. Here are several behavior types that could lead to aggressive biting:

- Anxiety and fear may be expressed by cowering, ears and head down, tail between the legs, as well as unwanted urination. These animals will likely bite once their flight distance is reached. Flight distance is characterized as the proximity a person or animal gets to another animal that causes a response which may include biting or fleeing.

- Aggression may be expressed by hissing, growling, exposed teeth, ears back, and the tail up or down. In cats, a wagging tail is a sign of discontent and aggression. Sometimes, these animals can be quite unpredictable when they strike.

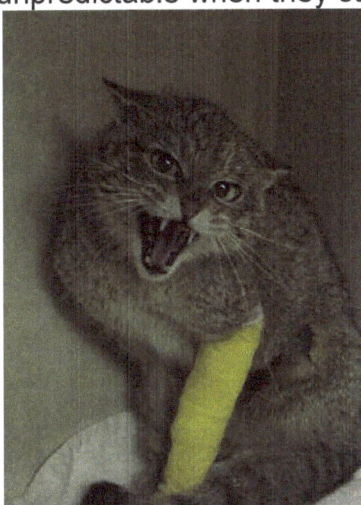

- Complacent animals tend to be unbothered by any manipulation. They will often wag their tails and behave happily. This can lead to complacency by the handler and potentially result in injury, if the manipulation suddenly becomes painful.

Animal perception is an important consideration for the animal handler. Animals have the ability to read emotions, including fear. Most handler injuries occur as a result of complacency or hesitation due to fear. Confidence and proper body language are essential when handling animals. Tone in communication and commands needs to be strong, but not overpowering. Predatory animals, like dogs and cats, may demonstrate dominance or submission when around other animals or animal handlers. Dominance can be used by the veterinary team to ensure compliance by the animals they are tasked to handle and restrain.

Types of Mechanical Restraint

Accessory restraint devices can be incredibly valuable when working with animals. These devices, not only protect the animal, but also provide protection for the handler. Here are some commonly used mechanical restraint devices:

- *Leash*-an easy way to control the movements of an animal; threaded through a fence, it can also secure an animal's neck.
- *Muzzle*-commonly made of fabric, it can be used to secure the mouth of an animal, reducing the possibility of bites.
- *Rabies pole*-useful for extracting animals from caves or small spaces, or for capturing animals from a safe distance.
- *Live trap*-useful for catching feral animals that are too fearful of being approached with a rabies pole.
- *Gloves*-an inexpensive means to avoid biting injuries to the hands; gloves tend to reduce one's dexterity when used.
- *Towel*-serves as a distraction as well as a hiding place for some animals; this can have a calming effect on some animals.
- *Bag*-useful for cat restraint, essentially preventing scratches by the claws.

Chemical sedatives and anesthetics can and must be used in some cases. Usually an animal must be restrained for an injection, however, some novel methods are also utilized:

- *Oral medications*-drugs are hidden in a food item and ingested by the animal.
- *Pole syringes*-essentially a syringe on the end of a pole, enabling injection from a safe distance.
- *Remote injection systems*-injection systems that use CO_2 driven rifles to shoot anesthetic containing darts at animals from a distance away.
- *Blow pipes*-anesthetic dart is blown through a pipe by lungs, this system has been largely replaced by CO_2 driven systems.
- *Induction chambers*-useful means of anesthetic induction in animals that cannot otherwise be safely handled.

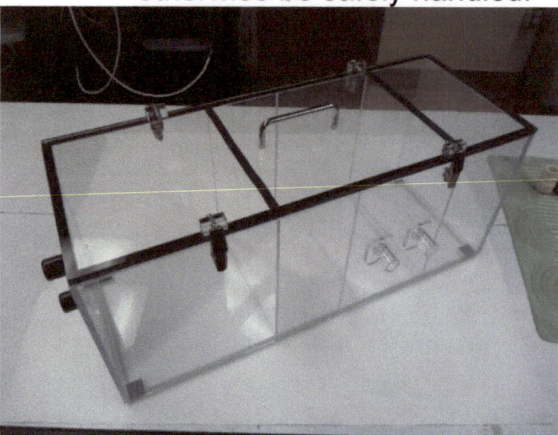

Figure 38: Induction chamber

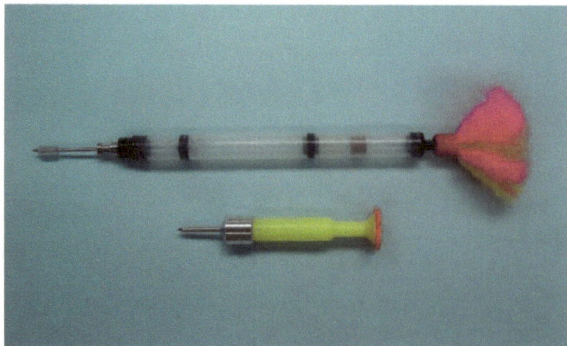

Figure 39: Remote injection darts

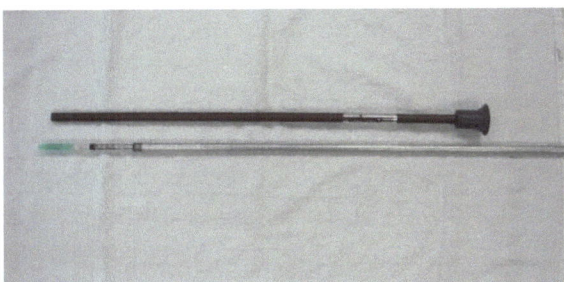

Figure 40: Blow dart pipe (top) and pole syringe

Lifting dogs and cats can be challenging and strenuous. Employing proper lifting techniques, whether it is a box or Boxer, is imperative. Boxes, however, do not move like a Boxer when being lifted; this adds a new dynamic to proper lifting. Here are some considerations when lifting animals:

- Bend with the knees, keep back straight; avoid leaning over the pet.
- Beware of the pet's back and abdomen; these areas may be painful.
- Cradle chest and hind when lifting the pet; this secures pet's limbs while protecting the abdomen.
- Get help if the pet is large, heavy, or squirmy.
- Properly restrain the pet's head so it does not hit exam table; use muzzle if necessary.
- Use the scruff for cat lifting; this usually has a calming effect, and tends to be safe for animal and handler.
- Keep a leash on all pets when possible; this prevents accidental escape if lifting goes wrong.

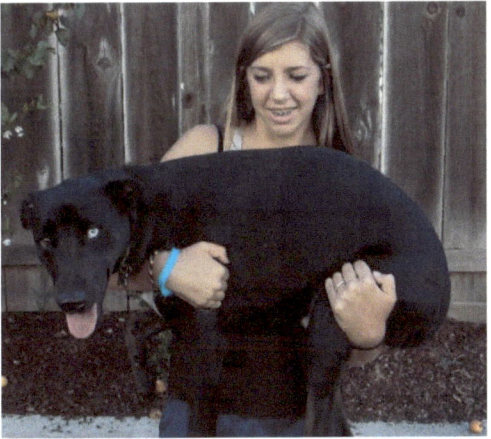

Figure 41: Proper holding of a dog

There are several reasons pets are restrained in a veterinary practice. Here are some examples:

- *Physical exam*-Patient may be standing or sitting; however, restraint of the head is important to ensure that the veterinarian does not get bitten while focusing on the exam.
- *ECG exam*-Patient is placed in right lateral recumbency or right side down.
- *Orthopedic examination*-Patient's limbs need to be evaluated, therefore, usually they need to be laterally recumbent or lying down on the side.
- *Anesthetic induction*-Patient is often sternal or sitting upright for induction with the front limb exposed for injection of anesthetic.
- *Catheter placement*-Patient is usually sternal with front limb exposed.
- *Radiography*-Lateral and ventral dorsal positioning is required to obtain both radiographic views.
- *Grooming and bathing*-pet needs restraint, usually minimal, while being washed and dried.

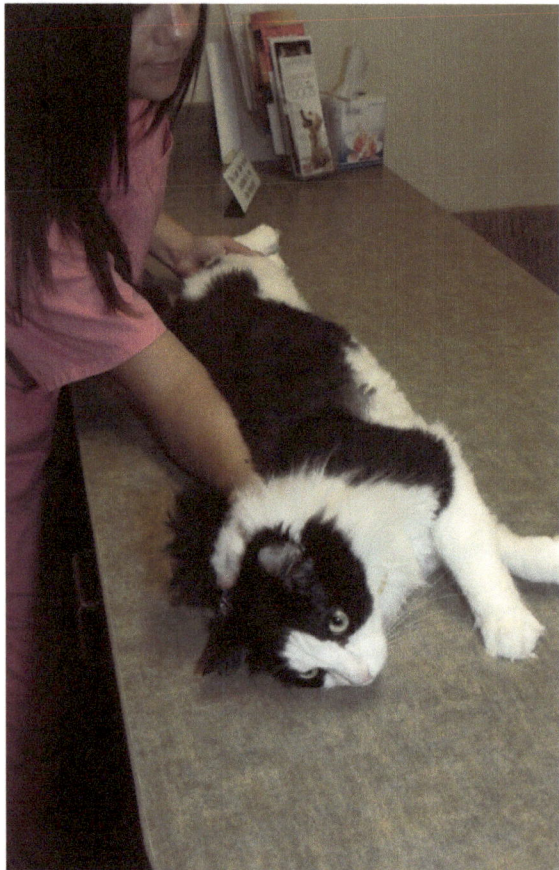
Figure 42: Cat stretch restraint

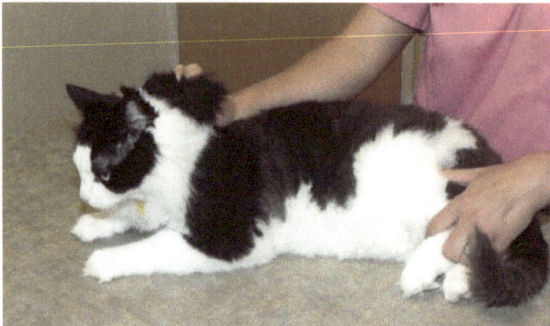
Figure 43: Cat scruff restraint

Phlebotomy or blood sample collection is a very important aspect of handling and restraint, as safe and effective blood collection is based on how well the patient is positioned. Positioning is usually based on several factors:

- *Phlebotomist preference*-some vessels are easier to obtain samples from, and some veterinary staff members may have preferred locations and positions for sample collection.
- *Patient*-some patients, like cats, may be more comfortable in lateral recumbency than sternal; others may be calmer while sitting.
- *Volume of blood sample needed*-larger blood volumes needed may require the use of larger vessels such as the jugular vein.

Commonly used phlebotomy locations and proper restraint techniques are described as follows:

The cephalic veins reside on the anterior (top) surface of both front limbs. These vessels are fairly robust in dogs; however, they can be more difficult to access in cats. These veins may be utilized in cases where a small sample is needed, or if the patient is medium to large in size. Here are the steps:

1. Place the patient in a sitting or sternal position.
2. Position yourself on one side of the patient.
3. Restrain the patient's head with one of your arms, and use the other arm to restrain the patient's opposing front leg.
4. Hold out the opposing leg, occluding the cephalic vein with your hand at the pet's elbow.
5. Roll your hand laterally (outward) putting tension on the cephalic vein.

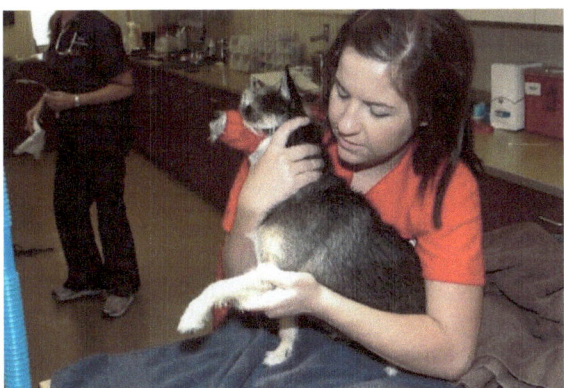
Figure 44: Restraint for cephalic venipuncture

The saphenous veins can be found on either side of rear limbs. These vessels are relatively small, and can be used in similar situations as the cephalic vein. The lateral (outside) saphenous vein can be readily seen in most shorthaired dogs. It runs in an upward direction from the anterior to posterior aspect of the rear limb above the hock joint. Here are the steps for the lateral saphenous vein:

1. Place the patient in lateral recumbency by carefully holding the head while pulling the legs away from you; this may require two people.
2. Take your front arm and rest it on the patient's neck, then restrain the pet's 'down side' front leg.
3. Take your other arm and occlude the saphenous vein just above the hock.

The medial saphenous vein is ideally used for cats. This vessel is more visible in cats than its lateral counterpart and restraint can be more successful. It is located on the inside of the rear legs, running most superficially from the stifle to the pelvis. Here are the steps for the medial saphenous vein:

1. Position the patient in lateral recumbency; if a cat, use the scruff for head restraint and the rear limbs for restraint of the body. Using these two points, the cat may be stretched along your

forearm; thus, limiting its ability to turn and move.
2. While someone, likely the phlebotomist, holds the 'down side' rear leg, position your hand across the 'down side' leg occluding the vessel. Use a karate chop hand position as it allows you to occlude the vessel while restraining and securing the abdomen and any fat bodies in the area.

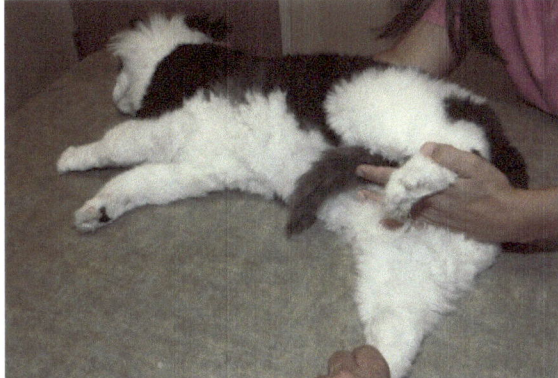
Figure 45: Cat restraint for medial saphenous vein access

The jugular veins are common sites for blood collection when larger volumes are needed. They are large vessels running on either side of the neck. They can usually be palpated within the jugular furrow; this is a channel that runs between the tracheal and the muscles of the neck. The jugular vein is usually orientated between the base of the mandible and the thoracic inlet at the sternum. Because of large amounts of fur, the jugular vein is often not visible to the naked eye, making the above landmarks important. Here are the steps for the jugular vein.

1. Place the patient in a sitting or sternal position.
2. Position yourself on one side of the patient.
3. Restrain the patient's head with one of your arms, and use the

other arm to restrain the patient's body; usually around the chest.

4. Lift the patient's head with your arm until its head is pointing toward the ceiling; this will expose the neck and jugular veins.

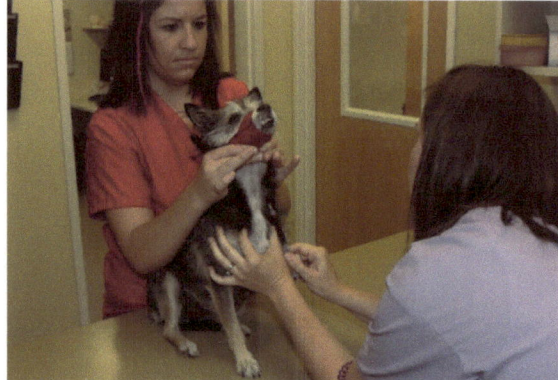
Figure 46: Restraint for jugular venipuncture

Other less commonly used blood collection sites may also be used. These sites are more commonly used in emergency situations where venous access is imperative.

- *The femoral veins* are located cranial and medial to the femoral artery on the inside of the rear legs. Access is made by splaying out the rear legs and palpating the femoral artery.
- *The coccygeal vein* is located on the dorsal aspect of the tail. This vein is more commonly used with livestock.
- *The lingual veins* are located under the tongue. These veins are useful in emergency situations with small or neonate patients.

Urinalysis is another situation where proper positioning is important for successful collection and safety to the patient. Urine samples can be collected using several methods. Urine collection from the ground or when the patient is urinating (free catch) usually requires little or no restraint. Sample collection by catheterization or cystocentesis, however, requires proper positioning and restraint.

- Urine collection by *catheterization* involves placement of a plastic tube into the urethra of the patient. This uncomfortable technique ensures a quality sample, free from most contaminants. In most cases, the patient is placed in lateral recumbency; the prepuce of the male is retracted exposing the penis, whereas a vaginal speculum is generally used in females. See figure 122.
- *Cystocentesis* is a method of urine collection where a needle is placed through the abdomen directly into the bladder. When done properly, this is a very aseptic and safe procedure. The patient is placed in dorsal recumbency; the area of the abdomen near the bladder is aseptically prepared. The needle connected to a syringe is punctured through the abdomen, then into the bladder. This method produces a nearly pristine urine sample with little to no contamination.

Other Handling Situations

One of the most common non-medical animal handling situations involves moving pets in and out of cages and kennels. In most cases, domestic animals are receptive to going into a cage or kennel. Some animals, however, may react poorly due to unfamiliar elements of a clinic setting. Here are some things to consider when moving an animal in and out of cages and kennels:

- The cage or kennel door is usually the only way in or out.
- Most animals, once released, will move away from the animal handler; this means when released into a cage or kennel, most animals will move to the back of the cage and not approach the door.
- Some animals, when cornered in a cage or kennel, will try to bite if approached; care should be taken when approaching animals in cages.
- Using your body to help block exit path will reduce the possibility of animal escapes.
- Having proper restraint equipment such as leashes, muzzles, or towels readily available will be beneficial if needed.
- Towels and other distractions can aid in the capture of a caged animal.

Anal glands are present in many species of animals including dogs and cats. These small scent glands are located on either side of the rectal opening. If the top of the rectum was the twelve o'clock position, the anal glands would specifically be located at four and eight o'clock.

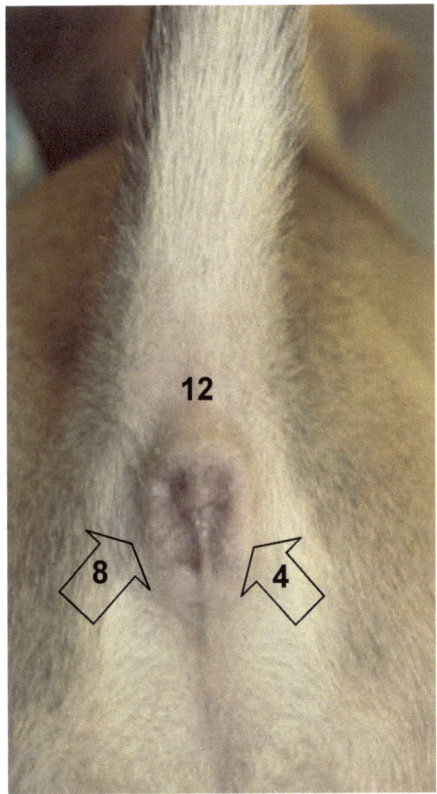

Figure 47: Location of anal glands based on a clock

The function of anal glands is to scent feces; olfaction is an important form of communication in many species. Anal gland secretions are very pungent. Under normal circumstances anal glands are expressed by passing feces, however, in some cases these glands may become impacted or the feces is not firm enough to express them. Anal gland impaction is more common in dogs. A characteristic of anal gland impaction is pet 'scooting'. If needed, the anal glands can be expressed. The pet should be restrained in a standing position; the head should be restrained, as the procedure tends to be uncomfortable. Using a latex glove, lubricate and insert the first finger into the pet's rectum. Position the finger cranial to the gland, and while putting pressure on the wall of the rectum, pull the finger outward until the gland is expressed. The process is repeated on the other side. In some cases permanent removal of one or both anal glands may be necessary if impaction becomes chronic.

Toenail trimming is a common procedure in veterinary clinics. Under normal circumstances, pet's nails are worn down by running on hard surfaces, digging and scratching. Long nails can be destructive to some floors and furniture; some cat owners even resort to declawing to contend with this problem.

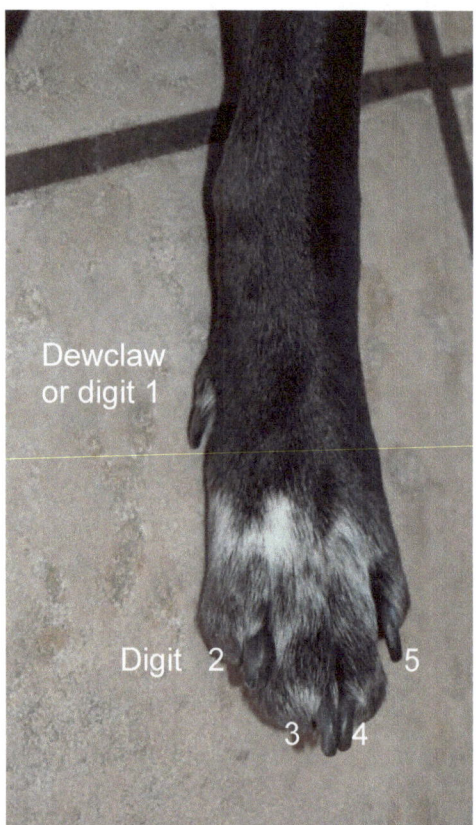

Figure 48: Digit numbering system of the left front foot of a dog; the dewclaws are always medial

The anatomy of the nail is similar in both dogs and cats; cats however, have retractable nails. The nail originates from the third phalanx of each digit. There are four digits on each foot, and in most cases, a single dewclaw on the medial aspect of each leg proximal to

the foot. The dewclaw is analogous to the thumb in humans. Under normal circumstances the nail length should be shorter than the tangential line from the surface of the toe pad.

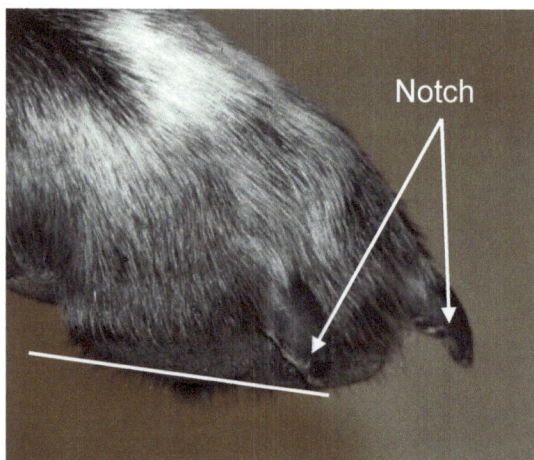

Figure 49: The nail length should be shorter than the tangent line made from pad; the notch is a good cutting point.

The nail is generally trimmed perpendicular to the nail above the tangent plane. There is generally a nail 'notch' present on the ventral or the underside of the nail. This can be used as a general reference point for trimming. The nail has a vascular supply also known as a 'quick', which is readily visible in pets with light colored nails. Locating the quick in pets with black nails can be challenging and may require small incremental cuts. Resco nail trimmers can be used for most nail trimming procedures and offer ease of use and a guillotine type cut. In the event that the quick is cut, several hemostatic powders such as Quick-Stop can be used to stop bleeding. Silver nitrate sticks can also be used, but tend to be staining to the skin.

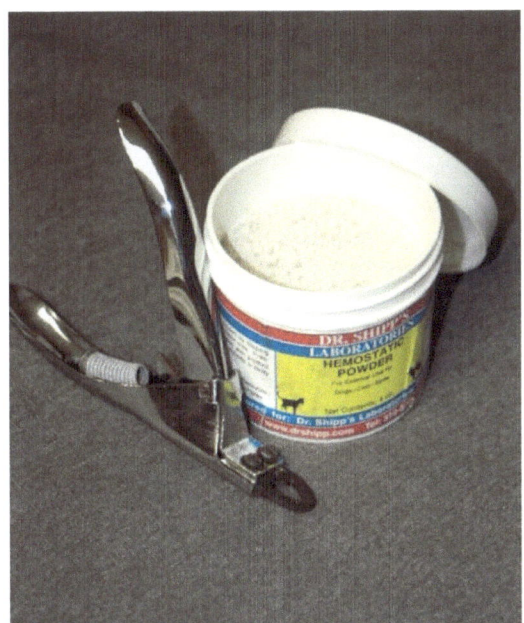

Figure 50: Resco nail trimmer and hemostatic powder

Ear cleaning is a necessary procedure for some pets. Bacterial and yeast infections, canal stenosis or narrowing, foreign bodies and parasites are reasons for ear cleanings at veterinary clinics. Some pets are predisposed to ear problems due to reduced airflow because of their large pinnas or hair filled ear canals. Symptoms of an ear infection include head shaking, scratching, excessive waxy debris and a pungent odor emitting from the canal. Ear cleaning products are designed to both break up wax and have drying properties so fluid does not persist in the ear canal. The ear cleaning solution is placed in the canal and filled; the solution may be warmed to reduce the sensitivity of a cold liquid being placed in the ear. Once filled, the base of the ear canal is gently massaged to loosen wax and debris within the ear canal. Care must be taken not to massage this area too vigorously, as facial nerve damage can occur. After massaging the ear canals, allow the pet to shake its head, thus forcing the solution and

debris out of the canals. This procedure is generally best done outside, or with the use of a towel drape to reduce the splashing of ear cleaning solution on walls and furniture. In some cases, a bulb syringe is used to flush the ear cleaning solution deep into the canal. This procedure may be uncomfortable to the pet, so care should be taken. After cleaning, gauze pads or cotton tipped applicators can be used to remove any residual debris from in and around the ear canal.

Routes of Administration

A route of administration is considered the path by which a drug, fluid, poison or other substance is brought into contact with the body. The route of administration is important when considering the action and quickness of activity of a drug. Some common routes used in veterinary medicine include:

- Topical
- Enteral
- Parenteral

Topical medications are generally given at or near where the action of the drug is desired. Examples include inhalational medications, eye and ear medications, and medications applied to the skin and mucous membranes.

Enteral medications are those given into the gastrointestinal tract and have systemic effects. Enteral medications include those given orally, rectally, or by gastric feeding tube.

Parenteral medications are those given by routes other than into the digestive tract. These medications are generally administered by injection. The most commonly used parenteral injection routes in veterinary medicine include:

- Subcutaneous
- Intramuscular
- Intravenous

Subcutaneous injections, often abbreviated SQ, are given in the space between the skin and muscle of a pet. The subcutaneous space in dogs and cats is abundant, and the area behind the neck called the 'scruff' is the most prominent. These injections tend to be the slowest in action of the above three, because drugs must be absorbed into the muscle before getting to the blood stream.

Intramuscular injections, abbreviated IM, are given directly into the muscle of the patient. These injections can be given into any muscle, but care must be taken to avoid vessels and nerves within the muscles. Because IM injections are given into vascular muscle, drugs get into the bloodstream more quickly than SQ injections.

Intravenous injections, abbreviated IV, are given directly into the vein of a patient. Drugs given in this manner have the quickest action because they are administered directly into the bloodstream.

Route	Location	Abbreviation
Intra-arterial	Artery	-
Intracardiac	Heart	IC
Intradermal	Dermis	ID
Intralingual	Tongue	-
Intraosseous	Bone	IO
Intraperitoneal	Abdomen	IP
Intrathecal	Spinal canal	IT
Intratracheal	Trachea	-

Figure 51: Less frequently used injection routes

How to Administer Topicals

Topical medications come in a variety of forms including ointments, creams, sprays and transdermal patches. These medications may include antibiotics or medications for pain and itch relief. Because topical medications are designed to be absorbed into the skin, gloves should be worn while applying these products. Additionally, Because of the potential for the pet to lick these types of medications, the use of an Elizabethan collar should be considered.

Ophthalmic medications usually come in two forms: drops and ointments. Ointments are more viscous and therefore tend to stay in the eye for longer periods of time. Eye drops need to be instilled more frequently than ointments. Care should always be taken not to injure the eye with the tip of the medication bottle. Holding the bottle, rest your hand on the patient's head and allow the drops or ointment to fall into the eye from above; avoid pointing the bottle directly at the eye.

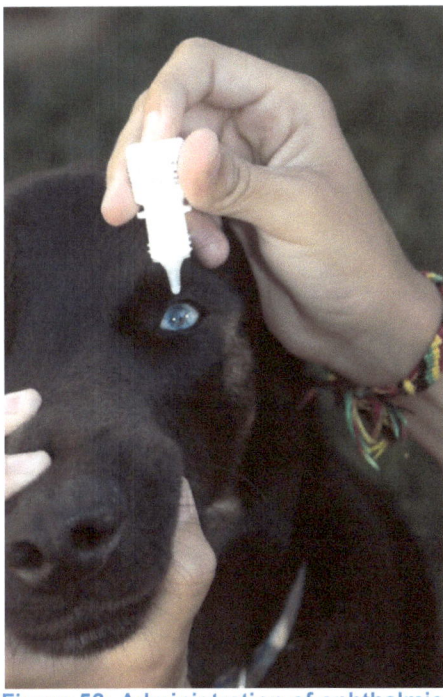

Figure 52: Administration of ophthalmic drops

Ear medications or otics, are generally solutions or viscous liquids designed to clean, dry, or coat the inner surfaces of the ear. Some of these products are used to treat infections and inflammation of the ear canal. After instilling the medication, gently massage the base of the ear to ensure that the medication gets effectively distributed within the ear canal. Horner's syndrome, a condition resulting in ptosis (drooping of the eyelid) from the damage of the facial nerve, can result if ear massaging is too vigorous.

How to Administer Enterals

Enteral medications come in a variety of forms including pills, capsules, chewables, liquids and suspensions. The easiest means of administering enteral medications is by hiding them in food items. Some medications even have palatable flavors in order to make medicating the pet easier. If these methods do not work, however, 'pilling' the pet may be necessary. Pet pilling involves getting the medication in the mouth and past the tongue. Doing this ensures that the pet receives the medication and it is not spit out. Effective pet pilling includes having the pet in a sitting position. Once sitting, your hand can be placed over the snout. Using the thumb, push in between the teeth to open the mouth. As you are opening the mouth, point the head upwards causing the mouth and esophagus to be in a straight line. Once the mouth is open, a pill may be given using two techniques.

1. Drop the pill in the mouth as far back in the throat as possible. If necessary, quickly push the pill as far past the tongue as possible with your finger or hand.

2. Using a pet piller, place the pill at the end of the device. Insert the piller into the pet's mouth as far back as possible, and then push the plunger on the piller. Pushing the plunger releases the pill from the piller.

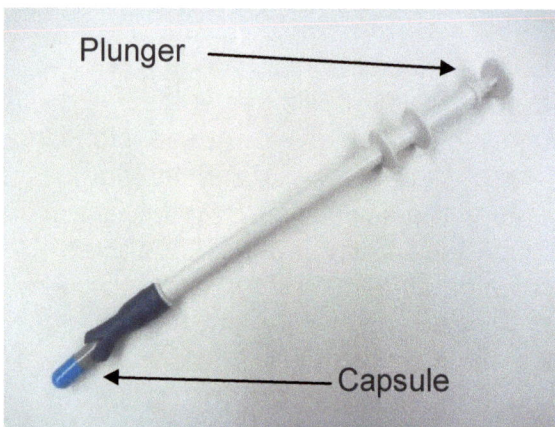
Figure 53: Pet piller with capsule

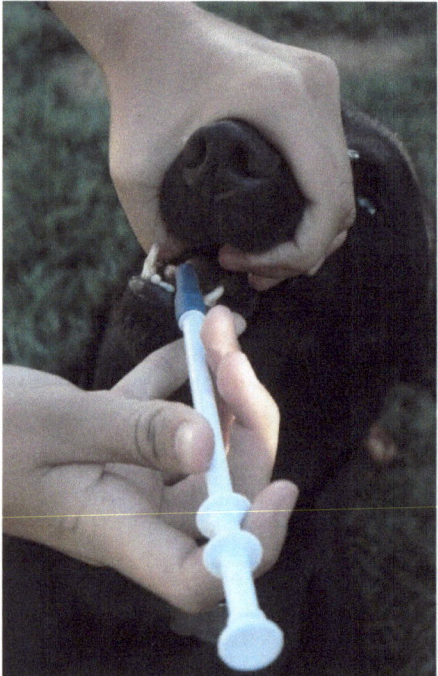
Figure 54: Pilling a dog

Because pets may not find oral medications palatable, the use of a flavor additive is sometimes used. These additives include liver, tuna, watermelon, and other more tolerable flavors. Drug compounding companies can improve the palatability of most medications by creating a flavored suspension. These suspensions must be shaken well to ensure that the medication is properly mixed.

Gavage tubes can be used to administer liquid medications to pets. These tubes are made of rubber, plastic, or metal, and are designed to be placed far into the mouth without necessitating the use of one's hand. Gavage tubes fit on the end of most syringes.

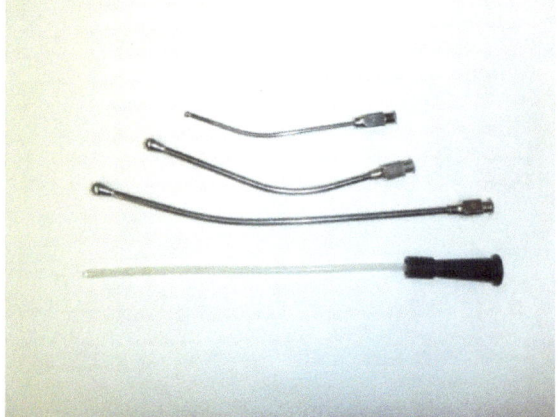
Figure 55: Metal gavage tubes (top 3), and plastic tube (bottom)

The challenges of pet pilling include personal injury from bites while administering the medications, traumatic hazards to the pet when using gavage equipment, and aspiration of medications into the pet's airway. Clients can be educated on the proper use, storage and administration of prescribed medications for their pet. In some cases, however, patients may need to be hospitalized in order to insure proper medication administration and compliance.

How to Administer Parenterals
Parenteral medications are generally used in the veterinary practice, whereas an oral version of the drug is sent home with the client if prescribed. This is because administration of parenterals involves the use of syringes and needles. Care should be taken when using syringes and needles, as inadvertent needle sticks from a drug

filled or contaminated syringe can be dangerous and potentially lead to infection.

The anatomy of a syringe:
- Barrel
- Plunger
- Units

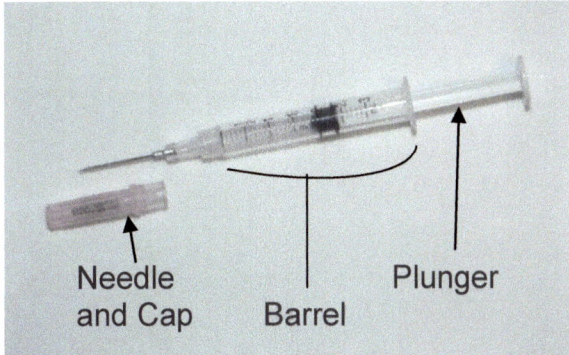

Figure 56: Parts of a syringe

Syringes come in a multitude of sizes and types; some are used for delivering small volumes, while others may be used for flushing of wounds. Some of the most common syringes in veterinary medicine include the insulin and tuberculin syringes, as well as the 3ml, 6ml, 12ml, 20ml and 60ml syringes.
Typically, insulin syringes are used by diabetic patient's in order to deliver exacting amounts of insulin. The measurements on the syringe are referred to as units. The syringes commonly hold 0.3ml, or 0.5ml, and usually have a 28 or 30 gauge wedged on needle.
Tuberculin syringes are slightly larger than insulin syringes and have increments in milliliters (ml). A variety of needle sizes can be used.
The most common syringe used for vaccinations in dogs and cats is the 3ml

syringe. Larger syringes (6ml, 12ml, etc.) are used for medication administration where volumes needed to be delivered exceed 3ml.

Syringe Units
Most syringes have units so exact amounts of the drug can be measured and delivered to the patient. The increments between numbers can vary, so careful determination of the value of each increment is important. For example, a three milliliter syringe (3ml) has numerical measures every one half milliliter. Between these numbers are small hash marks; in the case of the 3ml syringe, each hash mark equals 0.1ml. Therefore, when drawing up 0.7ml of a drug, the syringe plunger would be drawn back to the ½ ml (0.5ml) mark plus two hash marks.

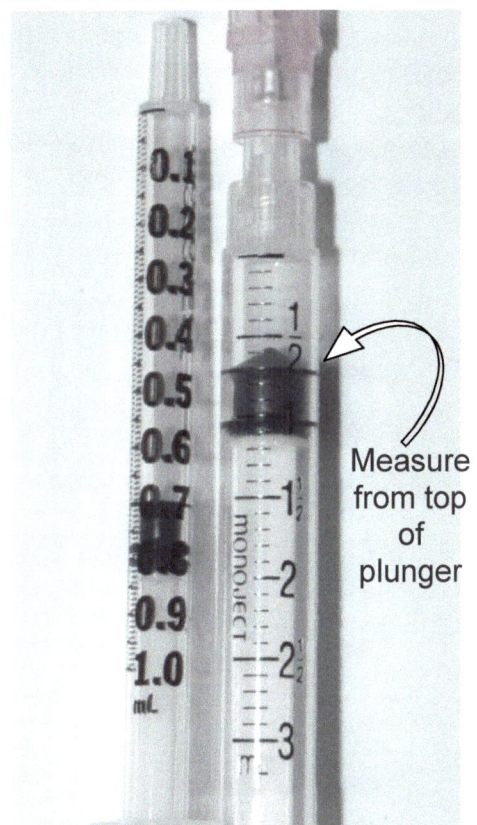

Figure 57: A 1ml (left) and 3ml syringe showing 0.7ml measured at the top of the plunger

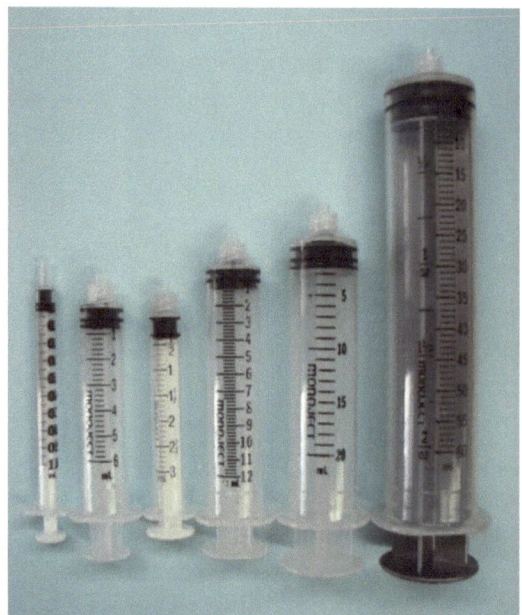

Figure 58: Assorted syringes

Syringes come with several types of tips; some are used for needles, while others are used for flushing and irrigation. Commonly used syringe tips found in veterinary practices include the Luer locking and tapered slip tips, the curved tip and the catheter tip syringes. Luer tips enable a needle to be wedged on to a syringe by friction, or locked in place by threads. Both types provide a leak free connection of the needle to the syringe. Curved tip syringes are often used for flushing and irrigating wounds. Catheter tip syringes are designed to accept a red rubber catheter. Uses include gavage feeding, gastric sample collection, and urinary catheterization.

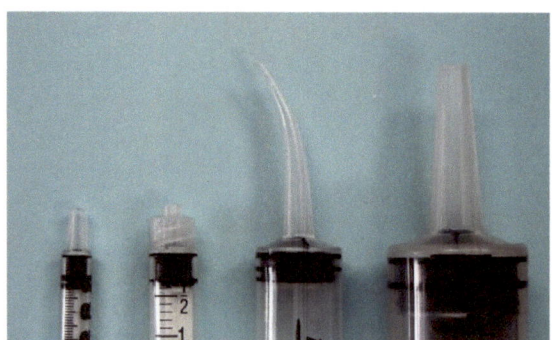

Figure 59: Syringe tips from left to right; luer slip, luer lock, curved and catheter tip

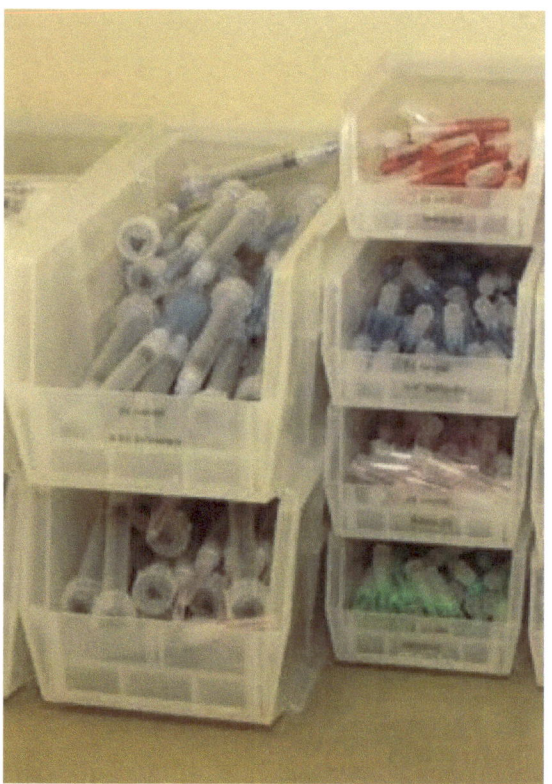

Figure 60: Syringes and needles. Note needles are color coded by size

The anatomy of a needle:
- Hub
- Shaft
- Tip/bevel

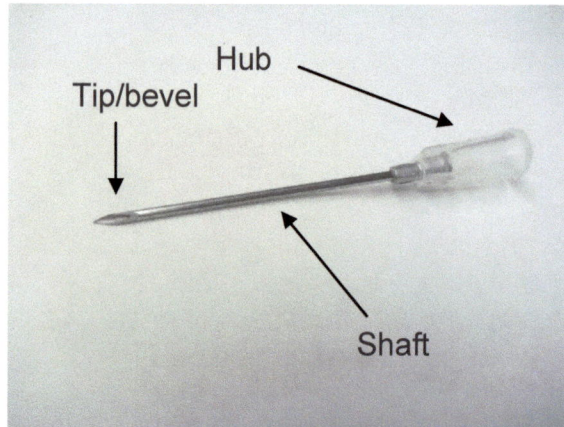

Figure 61: Anatomy of a hypodermic needle

Needle sizes vary in diameter and length. Needle diameters range from 30guage to 10guage. The gauge (ga) system, similar to how wire thickness is measured, uses a numbering system where the smaller the number, the larger the wire diameter. In this system, a 20ga needle has an outside diameter of 0.9mm and a 25ga needle has an outside diameter of 0.5mm.

The smaller the needle diameter, the longer it takes for fluid to pass through it.

Needle lengths range from 5/8 inches to 1½ inches, with 1-inch length being the most common. Longer needle lengths may be needed when injecting patients with thick skin or fur, or when samples are being taken from within the body cavity.

Other types of needles used in veterinary practices include:
- Blunt needle
- Spinal needle
- Butterfly needle

Blunt needles are useful as a small irrigation needle, or when flushing the eyes. These needles have a blunt tip, so there is minimal chance of causing injury to the patient.

Spinal needles are used for the collection of cerebral spinal fluid (CSF). These needles are usually 22ga to 18ga in diameter, and as long as 6 inches. These needles also contain a stylet that runs down the center of the needle. The stylet prevents material from clogging the lumen of the needle.

Butterfly needles are useful as a temporary infusion catheter, or used when giving injections to a fractious animal. Butterfly needles have small wings to hold while placing the needle; these wings also allow the needle to be secured to the patient. The needle is attached to a length of tubing that can be connected to a syringe. Once placed, a butterfly catheter will allow for patient movement without causing injury.

When selecting a needle size and length, it is important to consider the following:
- What size is the patient
- Where is the patient to be injected
- What is being injected

Smaller patients may benefit by the use of smaller needles. Injections may be uncomfortable, and using a smaller needle with these animals may reduce the discomfort. A larger patient may not respond to an injection no matter what needle size is used.

Injections into the subcutaneous space cause less discomfort than those into the muscle. Using a smaller gauge needle when giving IM injections may reduce the pain or adverse response the patient experiences.

Viscous fluids may not flow through a small diameter needle. Thick injectables like the antiparasitic medication, ivermectin, require the use of a 20ga or larger needle.

Tricks for syringe and needle use:
- Point the syringe up when drawing out medications from a bottle. Make sure the needle is below the fluid line of the bottle.
- Tap on side of syringe to get any air out of the syringe. Draw up more medication than needed initially.
- Inject a quantity of air into the bottle equal to the amount of medication needed. Air pressure in the bottle will force medication into the syringe.
- Use a new needle after drawing up medications. Needles dull easily.

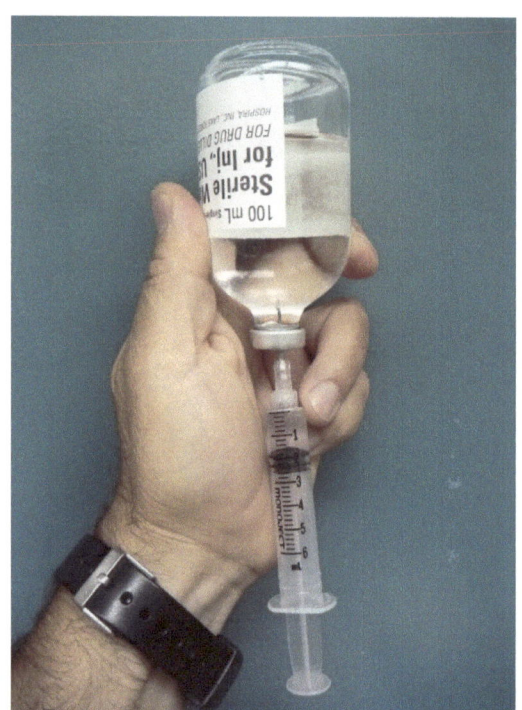
Figure 62: Proper technique for drawing injectable liquids into a syringe

Subcutaneous Injections

Dogs and cats have plentiful SQ injection sites; one of the most common is in the interscapular space behind the neck. This area provides abundant space for injection, as well as the safety of being out of biting reach from the patient. Restraining the patient will help to eliminate patient movement during the injection.

The skin at the injection site is lifted up with one hand and pulled away from the muscle creating a 'tent'. This tent creates a space between the skin and muscle known as the subcutaneous space.

The syringe is held with the other hand, and the bevel of the needle is positioned upwards. For consistency purposes, it is usually best to have the needle bevel upwards. The syringe and needle are then directed at a forty-five degree angle into the pocket created by tenting the skin. Once the needle is within the SQ space, pull back slightly on the plunger (aspirate) to ensure that a vacuum exists; there should be little to no free air present in the SQ space. If air enters the syringe when the plunger is pulled back, then the needle is likely not in the SQ space, and more likely has been driven through both layers of skin. If this occurs, pull the syringe and needle out and repeat the procedure.

Intramuscular Injections

Injection sites for IM injections in dogs and cats include the muscles of the front and rear limbs, as well as the lumbar muscles of the back. The rear legs are especially convenient because they are at a distance from the head of the patient (biting end) and the muscles are large. One concern about IM injections in the rear limbs pertains to the sciatic nerve. The sciatic nerve is a large nerve found deep in the muscles of the rear limbs. This nerve leaves the spinal cord and continues down the inside of the leg along the length of the femur. Injecting medication into the sciatic nerve can cause permanent nerve damage and should be avoided. Proper patient restraint will reduce the possibility of injury to muscle tissue or the sciatic nerve. In addition to nerves, muscles are highly vascular and contain many blood vessels. It is important not to give IM medications into a vessel.

Hold the limb being injected with one hand; if possible hold the muscle body being injected to ensure its location and stability.

With the needle bevel up, direct the syringe at a ninety-degree angle into the muscle. Injecting perpendicular to the muscle will make certain of where the needle is being placed and reduces the possibility of angling away from the desired location.

Once the needle has penetrated the muscle, pull back on the syringe plunger (aspirate) to confirm that the needle is not in a vessel. The presence of blood in the syringe after aspirating implies that the needle is in a vessel and should not be injected. Pull the syringe and needle out, and redirect to a new location.

Intravenous Injections

The most common IV injection sites on dogs and cats are the jugular, cephalic and saphenous veins. Proper restraint is very important when administering IV injections and its success is often based on the quality of the restraint. A struggling patient can lead to injury of its vessels, hematoma formation, or tissue damage due to paravascular administration of IV medications.
With one hand, stabilize the limb and vessel to minimize their movement. Use a tourniquet or the animal restrainer to hold off the vessel being injected. With the bevel of the needle pointing upward, approach the vessel with the syringe at approximately a thirty-degree angle. Aspirate the plunger of the syringe to ensure that the needle is in the vessel. Remove the tourniquet or have the animal restrainer release the vessel so medication can be administered. Infuse the medication slowly if indicated, watching for the formation of a hematoma or paravascular drug administration. If this occurs, stop injecting immediately.

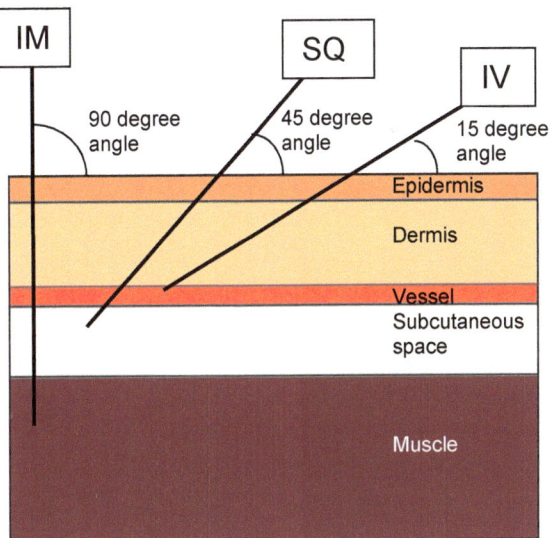

Figure 63: Injection angles

Medical Math

Medical math is an essential part of veterinary medicine. Whether it is calculating medicine doses or determining quantities of drugs needed, basic math skills are necessary. These skills include addition and subtraction of numbers, multiplication and division, as well as working with fractions, percentages, and decimals. Furthermore, the metric system is the fundamental measurement system in medicine and must be comprehended.

The Metric System
The metric system is a decimalized system of measurement used all over the world. The United States is one of a few countries not formally using the metric system. The main feature of the metric system is the use of decimal units and prefixes in powers of ten. For example, the meter, a unit of measure, can be converted to kilometers or millimeters by simply moving the decimal point, by a power of ten, to the left or right.

The US system of measure utilizes an array of conversion factors including the inch, foot, yard, and mile; the metric system functions to simplify those relationships. U

Measure	Basic unit	Abbreviation
Weight	Gram	g or gm
Volume	Liter	ℓ
Length	Meter	m

Table 10: Basic metric units used in medicine

Think of the metric basic unit as a root word. With any root word, changing the prefix changes the meaning of the word. For example, when the prefix *kilo* is added to the root word *gram*, kilogram is formed. A kilo is a factor defined to be 1,000, and hence, a kilogram becomes 1,000 grams. When kilo is applied to a meter, a kilometer is formed; a kilometer is equal to 1,000 meters.

Prefix	Symbol	Scale	Decimal
Kilo	k	Thousand	1000
Hecto	h	Hundred	100
Deca	da	Ten	10
Basic unit-no prefix	none	One	1
Deci	d	Tenth	0.1
Centi	c	Hundredth	0.01
Milli	m	Thousandth	0.001
Micro	µ	Millionth	0.000001

Table 11: Standard metric prefixes

Prefix	Factor	Relationship
Kilo (k)	1,000	1kg=1,000g
		1km=1,000m
Deci (d)	0.1	1dl=.1ℓ
Centi (c)	0.01	1cm=.01m
Milli (m)	0.001	1mg=.001g
		1ml=.001ℓ
		1mm=.001m
Micro (µ)	0.000,001	1µg=.000,001g
		1µm=.000,001m
		1µl=.000,001ℓ

Table 12: Commonly used metric prefixes

Metric Conversion
Using the metric prefixes, a number of grams, for instance, can be represented as kilograms or milligrams by simply moving the decimal point.

- 1g=1,000mg by moving the decimal point 3 places to the right, or multiplying by 1,000.
- 1g=.001kg by moving the decimal point 3 places to the left, or dividing by .001.

OR

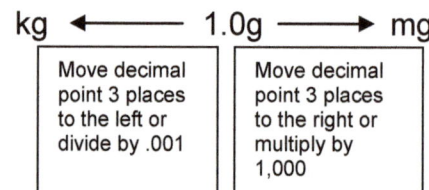

68

Using this method, 3.5g, for example, will be equal to .0035kg, and 3,500mg. To go from centimeters to millimeters, move the decimal to the right 1 place, micrometers to millimeters, move 3 places to the left, and so on.

k	h	da	Basic unit	d	c	m	-	-	μ
Move decimal point to the right 1 point → for each box when going from left to right									
←Move decimal point to the left 1 point for each box when going from right to left									
Note: each box represents a change of a factor of 10									

Table 13: Box diagram of decimal point changes for metric prefixes.

Metric Conversion to US Units

Several relationships between the metric system and the US system of measurement are necessary to convert between the two systems. One of the most important conversions in veterinary medicine is converting weight in pounds to kilograms.

- 1kg=2.2 pounds (lb)

This relationship implies that a patient's weight in pounds is roughly twice as much as that patient's weight in kilograms. Likewise, a patient's weight in kilograms is roughly half as much as their weight in pounds. Additionally, this relationship can be expressed as a fraction because of its equality. These fractions are useful for determining weight conversions algebraically.

$$\frac{1kg}{2.2lb} \quad and \quad \frac{2.2lb}{1kg}$$

Example 1: A patient weighs 22 pounds, how many kilograms does it weigh?

Mathematical solution:

$$22lb \times \frac{1kg}{2.2lb} = 22 \times \frac{1kg}{2.2} = \frac{22kg}{2.2} = 10kg$$

Note: lb's cancel out leaving kg's

Easy way to remember:

If you have pounds, divide by 2.2 to get kilograms.

Example 2: A patient weighs 6 kilograms, how many pounds does it weigh?

Mathematical solution:

$$6kg \times \frac{2.2lb}{1kg} = 6 \times \frac{2.2lb}{1} = 13.2lb$$

Note: kg's cancel out leaving lb's

Easy way to remember:

If you have kilograms, multiply by 2.2 to get pounds.

Example 3: A patient weighs 11 pounds, how many grams does it weigh?

Mathematical solution:

$$11lb \times \frac{1kg}{2.2lb} = 11 \times \frac{1kg}{2.2} = \frac{11kg}{2.2} = 5kg$$

Note: lb's cancel out leaving kg's

$$5kg \times \frac{1,000g}{kg} = 5 \times 1,000g = 5,000g$$

Easy way to remember:

a) If you have pounds, divide by 2.2 to get kilograms.

b) Once you have kilograms, move the decimal point to the right 3 places or multiply by 1,000 to get grams

Volumes of fluids need to be determined on a regular basis in a medical setting. All liquids, whether given orally or by injection, must be measured out accurately prior to administration. The preferred method of measure is the milliliter or cubic centimeter.

- 1ml=1cc

A milliliter is defined as 1 cubic centimeter of a liquid. This would be equivalent to a cube 1cm x 1cm x 1cm.

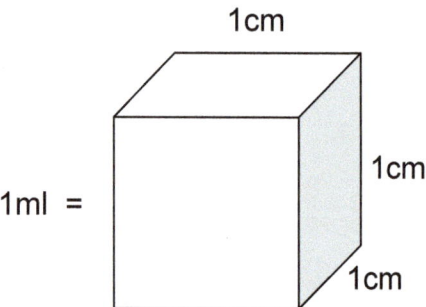

Geometric relationship between 1ml and 1cubic centimeter.

The US ounce can be converted to milliliters using the following conversion:

- 1 ounce=30ml

Algebraically this relationship can be expressed as:

$$\frac{1oz}{30ml} \quad \text{and} \quad \frac{30ml}{1oz}$$

Example 4: A patient is to be given 0.5 ounces of a medication, how many milliliters are given?

Mathematical solution:

$$0.5oz \times \frac{30ml}{1oz} = 0.5 \times \frac{30ml}{1} = 15ml$$

Note: oz's cancel out leaving ml's

Easy way to remember:

If you have ounces, multiply by 30 to get milliliters.

OR

If you have milliliters, divide by 30 to get ounces.

The conversion from milliliters to liters or microliters involves the moving of the decimal place based on the metric 'prefix'. For example:

0.015 ℓ	15ml	15,000µl
←	**Move 3 places**	→
Left		**Right**

Unit	Equivalent
1kilometer (km)	0.62 miles
1meter (m)	39.37 inches
1 centimeter (cm)	2.54 inches
1 liter (ℓ)	1.057 quarts
1 gram (g)	0.035 ounce
1 pound (lb)	16 ounces
1 US gallon	3.79 liters
1 tablespoon (TBS)	15 milliliters
1 teaspoon (tsp)	5 milliliters

Table 14: Other common conversions

The Units of Drugs

Drugs have units to indicate their *concentration*. These units are commonly in the form of milligrams (mg) for pill form medicines, and milligrams per milliliter (mg/ml) for liquids. The *dose* or amount of drug given to a patient is based on the concentration of the drug available. The dose is usually determined by the patient's weight in kilograms; the units for dose are generally expressed as milligrams (mg).

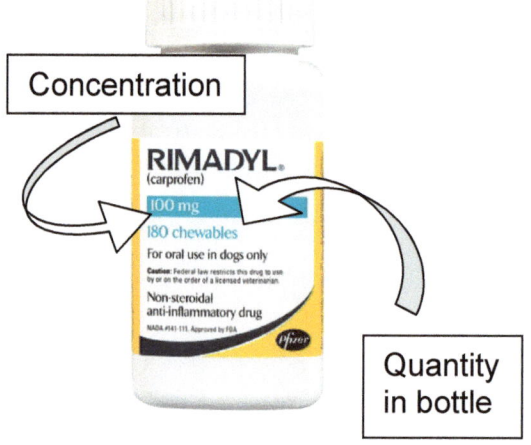

Concentration

Quantity in bottle

In the example of Rimadyl, each chewable tablet contains 100mg of carprofen; this is the concentration of the drug. The bottle contains 180 chewable tablets; this is the quantity of tablets in the bottle. If the patient were prescribed 200mg of carprofen, 2 chewable tablets would need to be administered.

> **Drug containers show the name of the drug, concentration of the drug, amount of pills or liquid in the bottle and the expiration date.**

The *dosage* of a medication is the recommended amount that the manufacturer suggests for the patient to produce therapeutic effects. The dosage, in most cases, is determined by the patient weight, and is generally expressed as milligrams of drug per kilogram (mg/kg).

Example 5: A 30 kg patient is prescribed the antibiotic amoxicillin at a dosage of 10mg/kg. The concentration of each capsule of amoxicillin is 100mg. What is the dose and quantity of drug administered to the patient?

Determine the dose by multiplying the patient's weight by the dosage.

$$30kg \times \frac{10mg}{kg} = 30 \times 10mg = 300mg$$

Note: kg's cancel out leaving mg's

Determine the quantity of drug administered by dividing the dose by the concentration of drug on hand.

$$\frac{300mg}{100mg} = \frac{3}{1} = 3 \text{ capsules}$$

Note: mg's and zeros cancel out

Easy way to remember:
'What you want, divided by what you've got', in this example, what you want is 300 and what you've got is 100,

so $\frac{300}{100} = 3$ capsules

Answer: The dose is 300mg, and (3) 100mg capsules will need to be administered.

Some drugs list their concentrations in percentages; these are often liquid medications. A percent solution indicates the composition of the drug in grams, in 100ml of solution. A percent solution is described by the following equation:

- % = g/dl (where a dl=100ml)

This equation can also be expressed as:

$$1\% = \frac{1g}{1dl} \times \frac{1000mg}{1g} \times \frac{1dl}{100ml} = \frac{10mg}{ml}$$

Example 6: What is the concentration of a 4% solution of injectable Thiopental?

$$4\% = \frac{4g}{dl} \times \frac{1000mg}{1g} \times \frac{1dl}{100ml} = \frac{40mg}{ml}$$

Note: grams(g) and deciliters(dl) cancel, leaving milligrams(mg) and milliliters(ml)

Easy way to remember: Move the decimal point 1 place to the right for all percent solutions.

Math Problems

Weight

A mouse weighs 18g. How many kg does it weigh?

18g x 1kg = 0.018kg
　　 1000g

A cat weighs 950g. How many Kg does it weigh?

A dog weighs 15,400g. How many Kg does it weigh?

A horse weighs1320 pounds. How many kg does it weigh?

A cat weighs 8.8 pounds. How many kg does it weigh?

A steer weighs 400kg. How many pounds does it weigh?

A dog weighs 10kg. How many grams does it weigh?

A dog weighs 20kg. How many pounds does it weigh?

A cat weighs 8kg. How many grams does it weigh?

A rat weighs 200g. How many kg does it weigh?

A rat weighs 200g. How many pounds does it weigh?

A rat weighs 200g. How many mg does it weigh?

A baby weighs 9lb 8oz, what is the weight in kg?

Measure

A tick measures 1cm in length. How many millimeters does it measure?

1cm x 10mm = 10mm
　　　 1cm

A parasite egg measures 6mm in length. How many centimeters does it measure?

A cat measures 20 inches from head to tail. How many centimeters does it measure?

A tumor measures 5cm x 4cm. How large is it in millimeters? How large is it in kilometers?

A red blood cell measures 7μm (micrometer or micron) in width. How many millimeters is this?

Volume

You have 9876ml of a liquid, how many liters is this?

9876ml x 1ℓ = 9.876ml or ≈9.9ml
　　　　 1000ml

You have 90ml of a liquid, how many liters is this?

You have 9ml of a liquid, how many liters is this?

You have 9 ℓ of a liquid, how many ml's is this?

You have 90 ℓ of a liquid, how many ml's is this?

You have 0.09 ℓ of a liquid, how many ml's is this?

You have 90ml of a liquid, how many ounces is this?

You need to dispense 50ml of liquid. You need a bottle at least this size.
   a. ½ ounce
   b. 1 ounce
   c. 1 ½ ounces
   d. 2 ounces

Dosage, dose, and quantity
A 10kg dog is to be given a 0.2mg/kg dosage of the antiparasitic drug ivermectin. What is the dose?
10kg x 0.2mg = 2.0mg
           kg

A 40kg dog is to be given a 0.1mg/kg dosage of the NSAID drug meloxicam. What is the dose?

A 20lb dog is to be given a 0.2mg/kg dosage of the antiparasitic drug ivermectin. What is the dose?

A 5lb cat is to be given a 15mg/kg dosage of the antibiotic enrofloxacin. What is the dose?

A 10kg cat is to be given a 10mg/kg dosage of the antibiotic amoxicillin. The concentration of the drug is 100mg. What is the dose and amount of drug to be given?

A 5lb dog is to be given a 12mg/kg dosage of the antibiotic enrofloxacin. The concentration of the drug is 22.7mg/ml. What is the dose and amount of drug to be given?

You are asked to give 1.5ml of the analgesic ketoprofen to a dog. The concentration of the drug is 100mg/ml. What is the dose given?

A 10lb cat is to be given the antibiotic clavamox twice daily for 10 days. The concentration of the drug is 125mg per tablet. The dose is 250mg. How many tablets must be sent home to fulfill the prescription?

A 50lb dog is to be placed on the antimicrobial metronidazole once daily for 30 days. The concentration of the drug is 50mg/ml. The dose is 125mg. What is the volume given each day? What is the total volume needed to fulfill the prescription?

Diseases of the Dog and Cat

Dogs and cats, just as humans, are susceptible to disease. These diseases may affect any body system of the pet, and may be the result of infectious, congenital, or degenerative processes. Some diseases can also affect specific breeds more frequently than others. Most breed-specific diseases have a genetic basis and may be passed from one generation to the next. Other breeds may have anatomical features that increase their predisposition to some diseases.

Here are several examples of conditions that may be seen in a veterinary practice and may be breed-specific.

Hip Dysplasia can affect large breed dogs, but some smaller breeds may be at risk. German shepherd and Rottweiler breeds are especially susceptible. Hip dysplasia is characterized by the abnormal articulation of the femur and acetabulum (hip joint). This may lead to osteoarthritis, which can be quite painful. Radiographs can be used to diagnose hip dysplasia, and are used by the Orthopedic Foundation of America (OFA) to certify that pets are free from this genetic disease.

Lipomas are benign fatty tumors common in most dog breeds. These tumors are usually of no consequence to the pet, but when they get large or ulcerated can be an esthetic problem. Lipomas can often be surgically removed in those cases.

Aural hematomas are a result of a ruptured blood vessel in one or both of the ears. This rupture may be caused by the excessive head shaking by the dog.

The structure of the canine earflap called the pinna, allows for the accumulation of blood within it. This blood filled pocket called a hematoma, generally does not resolve on its own and requires surgical intervention. Surgery involves lancing of the hematoma and suturing the skin so the pocket does not reform. Any dog can get an aural hematoma, but breeds with large pinnas such as the Cocker Spaniel and Bloodhound are more common.

Periodontal disease can affect any breed, but is more commonly seen in toy breeds such as the Poodle and Chihuahua. Periodontal disease is a symptom of swelling of the gingiva in the mouths of these pets. Gingival swelling, called gingivitis, leads to the destruction of tissues and ligaments surrounding the tooth root. This can lead to infection and tooth loss if left untreated.

Heart disease can affect any breed, but is more genetically common in breeds such as Boxers, some spaniels, and Great Danes.

Gastric dilatation-volvulus (GDV) or torsion is caused by the twisting of the stomach. This disease is common in very large dog breeds such as the Great Dane and Saint Bernard, and may be genetically linked. GDV is considered a life-threatening emergency and usually requires surgical intervention.

Diabetes mellitus affects both dogs and cats. Diabetes causes an unhealthy level of glucose buildup in the bloodstream; this is caused by the reduction or absence of insulin production by the body. If left untreated, Diabetes can lead to cataracts, neuropathy, and ketoacidosis. Diabetes mellitus is generally treated with insulin replacement injections and specific diets to help manage glucose levels.

Hyperthyroidism is caused by an overproduction of thyroid hormone by the thyroid glands. Thyroid hormone affects the function of most organs in the body. Common symptoms of hyperthyroidism include weight loss, increased appetite, increased drinking and urination, and increased activity. Hyperthyroidism is most commonly seen in older cats, and is rare in dogs. Treatment involves the use of thyroid suppressing drugs, radioactive iodine treatment, or surgical removal of the thyroid glands.

Glaucoma, a disease of the eye, can affect all breeds of dogs and cats. Glaucoma can be genetically predisposed for breeds such as cocker spaniel's, Australian shepherd's, and basset's, but can also affect other breeds as a result of cataracts, inflammation, or trauma.

Colitis is an inflammation of the colon leading to painful defecation, straining, and blood and mucous containing stools. Colitis can affect all breeds of dogs and cats at any age. Causes include inflammatory bowel disorders, dietary allergies, bacteria, parasites, stress or cancer. Treatments include the use of special diets and antibiotics.

Dermatitis affects more dogs than cats, and is characterized by any inflammation of the skin. The inflammation can be immune mediated, a result of external parasites, hormonal imbalances, bacteria, or fungi. The skin disease, seborrhea, is an inherited disorder. Some breeds such as the Sharpei, may be more susceptible to dermatitis because of their abundant skin and skin folds.

Vaccine Preventable Diseases

Canine Distemper is a contagious viral disease of dogs and wild carnivores. The virus is transmitted by infected body fluids including urine and feces. Unvaccinated puppies are at a higher risk of contracting the disease. Symptoms include fever, leukocytopenia, and encephalomyelitis.

Canine Parvovirus is a highly contagious viral gastrointestinal disease spread from dog to dog by contact with contaminated feces. Unvaccinated puppies are at a higher risk of contracting and dying from the disease than older dogs. Symptoms include vomiting, bloody diarrhea, fever, and dehydration. Treatment involves supportive care to counteract dehydration and electrolyte imbalances. Canine parvovirus is able to survive in the environment for many months, so proper decontamination is essential to reduce exposure to other animals.

Canine Adenovirus is an acute liver virus spread by infected feces, urine, blood, and nasal discharge. Symptoms include fever, loss of appetite, and liver disease symptoms such as jaundice. Most dogs recover without treatment.

Rabies is a viral disease of warm-blooded animals including dogs, cats, and humans. The disease is transmitted by the bite of an infected animal, and if left untreated, is almost always fatal. In the later stages of the disease, animals experience neurological signs, as well as hypersalivation and hydrophobia. Rabies is a Zoonotic disease.

Bordetella, or kennel cough, is a highly contagious airborne upper respiratory disease caused by one of several viruses or bacteria. Bordetella is transmitted through the air, so the disease spreads quickly in areas such as kennels that have a high density of animals. Symptoms include a dry hacking cough with or without the presence of a fever. Antibiotics and cough suppressants are used to treat symptoms.

Leptospirosis is a bacterial infection of dogs and humans. It is considered a Zoonotic disease, and transmission is usually the result of contact with water contaminated with infected animal urine. Symptoms include fever, headaches, vomiting, and diarrhea in people, and in dogs include liver and kidney damage, vomiting, fever, and lethargy.

Parainfluenza is a contagious viral respiratory disease characterized by coughing, nasal discharge, lethargy, and in some cases, pneumonia. Parainfluenza is sometimes mistaken for Bordetella infection.

Canine Influenza is a highly contagious viral respiratory disease. The virus can be spread by direct contact with respiratory secretions, or indirectly by contact with contaminated inanimate objects. Symptoms include coughing, nasal discharge, and in severe cases, fever and pneumonia.

Lyme disease is a tick borne bacterial disease affecting dogs and humans; it is a Zoonotic disease. Symptoms include fever, headache, and localized rash at the site of the tick bite. This is followed by joint aches, and central nervous system problems. Treatment involves the use of antibiotics.

Canine Coronavirus is a contagious gastrointestinal disease spread from dog to dog by infected feces. Originally thought to cause serious disease, it is now considered to have mild or no symptoms.

Giardiasis is an intestinal disease caused by a single celled protozoan. Diarrhea is the most common symptom, and treatment involves the use of antibiotics. Giardia can be diagnosed from a direct fecal evaluation or ELISA (enzyme-linked immunosorbent assay) testing to detect antibodies.

Feline viral rhinotracheitis (FVR) or feline herpesvirus, is a viral upper respiratory disease in cats. This highly contagious disease is transmitted by direct contact, and symptoms include coughing, fever, nasal discharge, sneezing, and conjunctivitis. In some cases pneumonia and death can occur.

Feline calicivirus causes respiratory infection in cats. Symptoms are similar to FVR, and although there is no primary treatment, antibiotics are used to treat secondary bacterial infections.

Feline panleukopenia, commonly called, feline distemper, is a viral infection caused by a feline parvovirus. Infection results from contact with infected bodily fluids, or from contaminated inanimate objects such as bedding and food dishes. Symptoms include fever, bloody diarrhea, dehydration, anemia and death.

Feline leukemia virus (FeLV) is a retrovirus spread from cat to cat by saliva, urine and bite wounds. FeLV can also be transmitted from an infected mother to kittens during nursing or in utero. FeLV causes immunosuppression in cats. Symptoms include inappetence, weight loss, poor coat condition, fever and eye problems. Prognosis is poor for FeLV cats. An ELISA blood test is used to determine possible infection, and is recommended prior to vaccination against FeLV.

Feline immunodeficiency virus (FIV) is similar to FeLV in its transmission and effects. FIV positive cats, however, may live healthy lives as carriers and transmitters of the disease. A blood test can determine the presence of FIV antibodies, but does not confirm infection. Vaccination may not be protective and will result in a positive antibody level if tested.

Feline infectious peritonitis (FIP) is a fatal disease of cats. The disease is transmitted by feces and contaminated surfaces. Of the 2 forms of FIP, the effusive or wet type is most common. An accumulation of fluid in the abdomen or chest is characteristic of the wet FIP, and results in dyspnea or difficult breathing. Other symptoms include inappetence, fever, weight loss and diarrhea. Treatment usually involves relieving symptoms and removing the ascites or fluid, but prognosis still remains very poor.

Immunology and Vaccines

The primary role of the immune system is to protect the body from invading microorganisms and foreign substances. The immune system functions to recognize the difference between the body's own cells and those that are 'non-like'. These foreign substances stimulate the immune system to react. These pathogens, if not eliminated, can lead to disease. Diseases include those mediated by viruses, bacteria, fungi and parasites. Tumor cells can also be destroyed by the immune response if they are identified as 'non self'. The immune system deals with these intruders, called antigens, by the use of the body's leukocytes or WBC's. These cells identify, ingest, or produce antibodies in response to invading antigens. An antibody, also known as immunoglobulin, can bind to an antigen so that it may be recognized by the body. These antibodies are produced by several mechanisms.

Passive antibodies are acquired from one's mother. These antibodies can be transferred to the unborn fetus while in the placenta, or when nursing immediately after birth. Colostrum, or first milk, is a form of milk produced by the mammary glands and is rich in maternal antibodies.

Active antibodies are acquired as a result of vaccination. Vaccines are designed to generate an antibody reaction by the body in the presence of an introduced antigen. These antigens generally do not lead to disease, but instead produce a body defense for subsequent exposures.

Natural exposure of antigens causes a natural immune response. Exposure to a live pathogen can lead to disease, but can also create an immunological memory for future exposures. Vaccination is an effective way to prevent infection and disease. Vaccines generate an immune response by the body, as well as specific antibody production. Vaccines are usually given in an initial series, followed by regular boosters. By doing this, the body can remain familiar with the antigen, and respond with antibodies quickly.

Several vaccine types are utilized in veterinary medicine. A vaccine contains an element that resembles the disease-causing organism, but often contains weakened or killed forms of the antigen. *Killed vaccines* contain antigens that have been destroyed by chemical or thermal processes. The body can still recognize the 'dead' components and generates an effective antibody defense. Some allergic reactions can be seen with killed vaccines due to the amount of antigen needed for an effective immune response. Killed vaccines have a lower duration of immunity and usually require an adjuvant. Adjuvants help stimulate the immune response, but may lead to additional local allergic reactions. *Modified live vaccines* contain antigens that have been attenuated or weakened to prevent the likelihood of causing disease. These vaccines generally provide a superior immune response because the intact pathogen is present. They usually require no adjuvant. *Recombinant vaccines* use live-vectored poxviruses to provide the vehicle for immune response. A piece of poxvirus gene is replaced by one or more pathogen genes. These vaccines are free from adverse effects, stable and nonadjuvanted. These vaccines also provide strong antibody response and immunity.

DNA vaccines use a small piece of bacterial DNA that has been genetically engineered to produce antigen proteins from a pathogen. These foreign proteins trigger an immune response. DNA vaccines are gaining popularity, and several vaccines including a canine melanoma vaccine are being used.

Vaccination schedules for puppies and kittens are based on the decreasing levels of maternal antibodies. Vaccine series are initiated around the time that passive immunity is easing. After receiving a vaccination, the immune system responds to the foreign substance by producing antibodies. This antibody response is rapid, with a significant amount of antibody production. In the absence of additional antigen, the antibody level slowly drops. When the next vaccination occurs, a heightened antibody response occurs; this increased response is due to the immune systems recognition of the antigen as a result of the previous vaccination. When the final vaccination is given, the antibody response and levels respond even quicker and with higher amplitude.

Figure 64 shows the antibody response to a vaccination series given at 8, 12, and 16 weeks of age. The amplitude of antibody levels increases after each vaccine is given. The series is started around the time when maternal antibody levels are depleting.

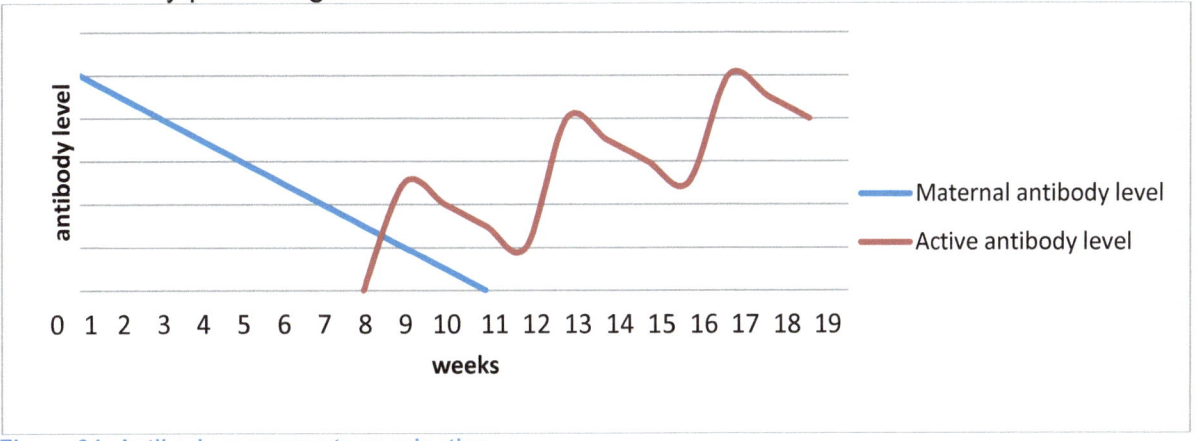

Figure 64: Antibody response to vaccination

Adult dogs and cats that have never been vaccinated are typically given a series of two vaccines approximately 3-4 weeks apart. This produces a similar antibody response as seen in figure 7, but because the immune system is more mature, a third vaccine is generally not necessary.

Rabies vaccination in dogs is mandated by State law; currently cats are not required to be vaccinated. The vaccination schedule for dogs involves an initial vaccine given at 4 months of age (16 weeks), a booster at 1 year, then subsequent vaccinations every 3 years.

Puppies and Kittens	8,12, and 16 weeks, or every 3-4 weeks until at least 16 weeks of age
Adult Dogs and Cats	2 vaccines 3-4 weeks apart

Figure 65: Initial vaccine schedules based on age

1.

In 2006, the American Animal Hospital Association released new guidelines for pet vaccinations. AAHA recognized that many vaccines, once administered, had greater protection for longer periods of time than once thought. Many vaccines historically given on an annual basis were found to be effective after several years. Additionally, AAHA reclassified the importance of vaccines based on disease prevalence and whether an individual pet may be in a high-risk group. The major changes included:

- Decreasing vaccination frequency to every 3 years in many cases
- Defining Core and Non-core vaccines
- Defining vaccines that are not recommended

Core Vaccines are those that protect pets from diseases that are endemic to a region, those with potential public health significance, those that are required by law, those that are highly infectious, and those that pose a risk of severe disease. Core vaccines have demonstrated efficacy and safety and exhibit a high enough level of patient benefit and low enough level of risk to justify their use in the majority of patients.

Non-core vaccines are those that fit any of the following criteria:

- Targeted for diseases that are of limited risk in the region
- Protects against diseases that present less severe threats to infected patients
- Have a benefit/risk ratio that is too low to justify the use of the product in all circumstances

- Lacks adequate scientific information to fully evaluate the safety and/or efficacy of the product

(Core/non-core vaccine information taken from AVMA vaccination principles, revised April 2007)

Canine vaccinations-Core Vaccines
- Canine Distemper
- Canine Parvovirus (MLV)
- Canine Adenovirus CAV-2 (MLV)
- Rabies

Canine vaccinations-Non-core Vaccines
- Bordetella
- Leptospirosis
- Parainfluenza
- Influenza
- Distemper-measels
- Lyme disease

Canine vaccinations-Not Recommended
- Coronavirus
- Giardiasis

Canine vaccinations-No Position
- Rattlesnake

Feline vaccinations-Core Vaccines
- Feline viral rhinotracheitis-feline herpesvirus
- Calicivirus
- Panleukopenia
- Rabies

Feline vaccinations-Non-core Vaccines
- FeLV
- FIV
- Bordetella

Feline vaccinations-Not Recommended
- FIP
- Giardiasis

2006 AHAA Canine Vaccination Guidelines					
Vaccine	Recommendation Core/non-core	Vaccine type	Puppy vaccination	Adult vaccination	Revaccination (Booster)
Canine Distemper	core	MLV	a minimum of 3 doses every 3-4 weeks until 16 weeks (ex. 8, 12, and 16 weeks)	2 doses 3-4 weeks apart. 1 dose is considered protective	all puppies should receive a 1 year booster, followed by every 3 year boosters
Canine Parvovirus	core	MLV	a minimum of 3 doses every 3-4 weeks until 16 weeks (ex. 8, 12, and 16 weeks)	3 doses 3-4 weeks apart. 1 dose is considered protective	all puppies should receive a 1 year booster, followed by every 3 year boosters
Canine Adenovirus	core	MLV	a minimum of 3 doses every 3-4 weeks until 16 weeks (ex. 8, 12, and 16 weeks)	4 doses 3-4 weeks apart. 1 dose is considered protective	all puppies should receive a 1 year booster, followed by every 3 year boosters
Rabies	core	Killed	administer 1 dose as early as 3 months of age; state requirements may vary	administer a single dose	a second vaccine is administered at 1 year of age or 1 year from initial vaccination. Booster vaccines are administered every 3 years [(based on using 3 year rabies vaccine) 1 year vaccine available]
Bordetella	non-core	killed	administer 1 dose at 6-8 weeks and 1 dose at 10-12 weeks of age	2 doses 2-4 weeks apart	annually, more for high risk animals
Bordetella	non-core	Live avirulent-intranasal	administer 1 dose as early as 3 weeks of age, a second dose should be given 2-4 weeks after the first	a single dose	annually, more for high risk animals
leptospirosis	non-core	Killed	administer 1 dose at 14 weeks and 1 dose at 14-16 weeks of age. For optimal response, do not administer before 12 weeks of age	2 doses 2-4 weeks apart	annually, vaccines should be restricted to use in areas where risk has been established
Parainfluenza	non-core	MLV	administer at 6 weeks, then every 3-4 weeks until 12-14 weeks of age.	a single dose	a booster at 1 year of age, followed by every 3 year boosters
Influenza	non-core	Killed	2 doses given 2-4 weeks apart after 6 weeks of age	2 doses given 2-4 weeks apart	annually
Distemper-measles	non-core	MLV	only 1 dose given between 4 and 12 weeks of age	never indicated for animals older than 12 weeks	never indicated for animals older than 12 weeks
Lyme disease	non-core	Killed	initial dose at 9 or 12 weeks of age, followed by a second dose 2-4 weeks later	2 doses 2-4 weeks apart	annually only for dogs with known high risk of exposure
Rattlesnake	no position	Toxoid	2 doses 1 month apart, given as early as 4 months of age	2 doses 1 month apart	annually, usually before rattlesnake season
Corona	not recommended	Killed and MLV	Frequency and severity of known clinical cases does not justify vaccination		
Giardia	not recommended	Killed	The vaccine may prevent oocyst shedding, but does not prevent infection		

2006 AHAA Feline Vaccination Guidelines					
Vaccine	Core/non-core	Vaccine type	Kitten vaccination	Adult vaccination	Booster
Feline Herpesvirus (FVR)	Core	MLV	a minimum of 3 doses every 3-4 weeks until 16 weeks (ex. 8, 12, and 16 weeks)	2 doses 3-4 weeks apart	a booster at 1 year of age, followed by every 3 year boosters
Feline Calicivirus	Core	MLV	a minimum of 3 doses every 3-4 weeks until 16 weeks (ex. 8, 12, and 16 weeks)	2 doses 3-4 weeks apart	a booster at 1 year of age, followed by every 3 year boosters
Feline Panleukopenia	Core	MLV	a minimum of 3 doses every 3-4 weeks until 16 weeks (ex. 8, 12, and 16 weeks)	2 doses 3-4 weeks apart	a booster at 1 year of age, followed by every 3 year boosters
Rabies	Core	Killed and Recombinant	administer 1 dose between 12 and 16 weeks of age	administer a single dose	a second vaccine is administered at 1 year of age or 1 year from initial vaccination. Booster vaccines are administered every 3 years [(based on using 3 year rabies vaccine) yearly with recombinant vaccine]
FeLV	non-core	Killed and Recombinant	2 doses 2-4 weeks apart before 16 weeks of age	2 doses 2-4 weeks apart	annual boosters based on risk
FIV	non-core	Inactivated dual subtype	May not protect against all FIV subtypes, risks and benefits should be evaluated before use		
Bordetella	non-core	MLV-intranasal	Could be used for young cats in high risk exposure environments, risks and benefits should be evaluated before use		
FIP	not recommended	MLV-intranasal	Vaccine efficacy is questionable, and duration of immunity is short. Risks are greater than incidence of FIP		
Giardia	not recommended	Killed	The vaccine may prevent oocyst shedding, but does not prevent infection, and may induce vaccine-associated sarcomas		

Vaccination Use and Administration

Vaccines are commonly packaged in single dose containers or in multi-dose drums. Additionally, some vaccines are premixed and ready for use, while others require mixing prior to use. Vaccines require proper handling and storage in order to maintain their potency; they must be refrigerated at temperatures ranging from 35-46 degrees Fahrenheit. Vaccines should be immediately used once removed from the refrigerator and prepared. Two component vaccines, those that need to be mixed, generally have a liquid aliquot or diluent and a dry lyophilized component. The diluent is drawn up with a syringe and inserted into the lyophilized component. After mixing, the vaccine is ready to be administered.

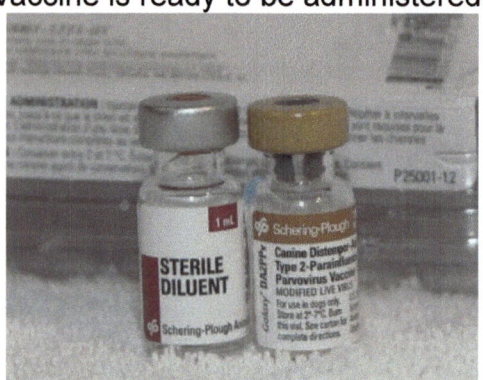

Figure 66: Two component vaccine, Diluent (left) and lyophilized aliquot

Most vaccines require the administration of a specific volume; usually 1 milliliter. The dose is the same for all sizes of animals and usually no adjustment in dose is made for very small pets. Vaccines are usually delivered by the following routes based on the vaccine type and manufacturer's recommendation.

- Subcutaneous
- Intramuscular
- Intranasal

Considerations for Administration

Vaccines can usually be safely and conveniently administered in the scruff area of most pets, but multiple sites may be needed if additional vaccines are given.

Site preparation is generally not necessary, but some veterinary staff may apply alcohol prior to administration of vaccines.

Hypodermic needles dull easily; preparing a vaccine can blunt the tip of a needle. The use of a new needle, after preparing a vaccine, may help make administration easier and less painful to the patient.

Twenty-two gauge needles are commonly used to administer vaccines. Smaller gauge needles may be beneficial in smaller pets; this may reduce the pain associated with the injection. The rate of injection, however, will likely be slower with smaller bore needles. This may be a disadvantage if the patient is fractious.

Risks of Vaccination

Adverse vaccine reactions can occur in dogs and cats; the risk of vaccination is relatively small compared to the risk of disease the vaccines prevent.

Anaphylaxis is a rare, life-threatening, allergic reaction to something ingested or injected. Vaccine administration can lead to anaphylaxis. The most common symptoms include vomiting, diarrhea, shock, seizures and in some cases death. Additionally, there may be local site reaction, facial swelling, or hive-like bumps. Anaphylaxis is more likely to occur with the use of killed vaccines, and those that use adjuvants.

Feline vaccine associated fibrosarcoma can occur in cats after the administration of vaccines containing adjuvants. Adjuvants like, aluminum hydroxide, stimulate the body's immune response and creates a local reaction at the vaccine site. Unfortunately, in some cases, tumor formation can occur. Sarcomas are aggressive, highly invasive malignant tumors that usually require surgery, chemotherapy and radiation therapy to eradicate. In cats, tumor formation usually occurs at the site of vaccine administration; this is commonly at the scruff of the neck. Unfortunately, these tumors can be difficult to remove, and their recurrence at the surgical site is common. After the recognition of the association of vaccination and sarcoma formation, recommendations regarding vaccine placement were made. It was concluded that in the event of sarcoma formation, removal of the animal's limb would be more successful than an attempted removal at the scruff. Furthermore, by specifying vaccination sites, it could be easier to determine the causative factors involved with tumor formation. As a result, the following vaccination placement guidelines for cats were made.

- FVRCP combo vaccine-given over the right shoulder
- Feline leukemia vaccine- given subcutaneously in the left rear limb
- Rabies vaccine-given in the right rear limb

Parasitology

Parasitology is the study of parasites, their hosts and their life cycles. One of the goals of animal parasitology is to protect animal health and prevent transmission to humans; thus, protecting human health. A parasite is generally thought of as an organism that benefits at the expense of another organism, or host. Endoparasites live inside the host, whereas, ectoparasites live on the outside of the host. In some cases, parasites utilize vectors to access the host. Some parasites have complex lifecycles involving more than one host. A parasite life cycle may include egg, cyst, larval, nymph and adult stages. Adult parasites, such as fleas and worms, are large and can be easily seen, whereas, their eggs may require the use of a microscope to visualize.

Parasites are found in most areas of the host's body including the:

- Oral cavity
- Esophagus
- Stomach
- Intestines
- Internal organs
- Skin
- Eyes
- Ears
- Brain

Major Classes of Parasites
Protozoa

- Single celled parasites that infect the intestinal tracts of animals. This group is referred to as the coccidians.

Helminths

- Multicellular parasites that include Nematode, Cestode and Trematode worms. The life cycle includes an egg and larval or 'worm' stage.

Arthropods

- Invertebrate parasites that include insects and arachnids.

Type	Class	Genus	Also known as:
Protozoa	Coccidia	Isospora Eimeria Toxoplasma Sarcocystis	
Helminth	Nematodes	Toxocara Ancylostoma Strongyloides Trichuris	Roundworms Hookworms Threadworms Whipworms
	Cestodes	Taenia	Tapeworms
	Trematodes		Flukes
Arthropod	Insects		Flies Fleas Lice
	Arachnids		Ticks Mites

Table 15: Common Types of Parasites

Sizes of Parasites

Parasites range in size dramatically, but most require the use of a microscope to be visualized. The micron (μm) is a commonly used unit of measure for these microscopic organisms. Most particles and organisms larger than about 20μm can be visible by the human eye, and include some large endoparasites eggs and most ectoparasites.

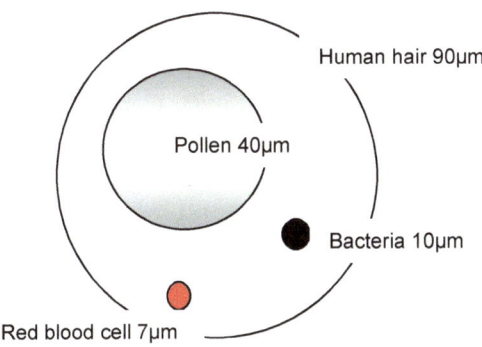

Figure 67: Comparison of size of pollen, bacteria, and red blood cell, relative to a human hair

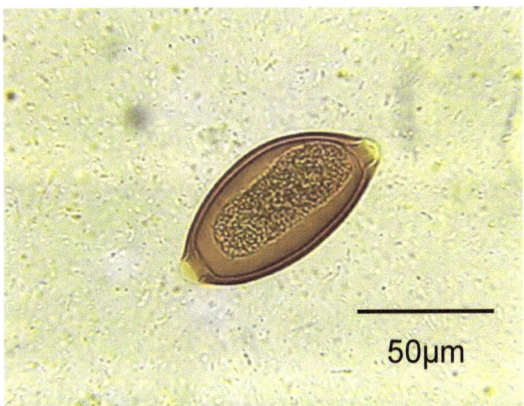

50μm

Figure 68: Whipworm (trichuris) egg approx. 35x90μm

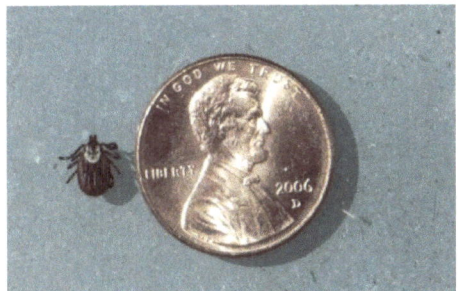

Figure 69: Adult tick approx. 4,000μm

Diagnostic Techniques

The most common type of parasite evaluation is the fecal analysis. Due to the potentially infectious and zoonotic nature of feces, proper safety techniques must be employed.

When working with fecal samples, veterinary staff members should wear protective latex gloves as well as eye protection. Refrain from eating and drinking while working with laboratory samples such as feces.

Several techniques are utilized when evaluating fecal samples for parasites; these include the following:

- Direct smear
- Floatation
- Centrifugal

The *direct smear* method requires a fresh fecal sample. In most cases the sample is acquired directly from the pet with the use of a fecal loop. The sample is placed on a microscope slide and a drop of normal saline is used to put the sample into solution. The sample is immediately evaluated with a microscope. Direct fecal smears are useful for identifying fragile parasites that may not be observed with other diagnostic techniques.

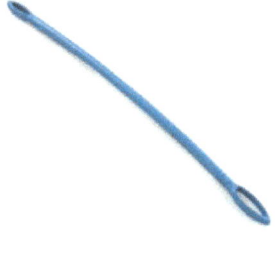

Figure 70: Fecal loop

The *fecal floatation* is the most common and convenient method of fecal analysis. Feces are placed into a specially designed plastic fecal container; this can be collected by the pet owner before arrival to the veterinary practice. The sample is diluted with a hypertonic solution such as zinc sulfate. The fecal container has an insert that allows for easy mixing of the sample. After mixing, the container is filled until a meniscus is created. A meniscus is created as a result of the cohesive property of water. It appears as a rounded surface at the top of the fecal container. A microscope cover slip is placed on the meniscus and allowed to sit for approximately 15 minutes. The hypertonic solution causes small, light particles, including parasite eggs, to float to the top of the container and adhere to the cover slip. The cover slip is then removed and placed on a microscope slide for evaluation.

The *centrifugal method* is similar to the floatation method except that the sample is placed into a centrifuge after being mixed with a hypertonic solution. Once spun, the resultant fecal pellet is evaluated under the microscope.
A paper cup or coffee filter may be used to filter large materials such as plants and debris from the fecal sample prior to evaluation.

The Microscope

The use of a microscope is essential when evaluating fecal samples. Microscopes are expensive, specialized and intricate pieces of equipment. The fragile optics can be easily damaged if improperly used. Care must be taken when working with microscopes.

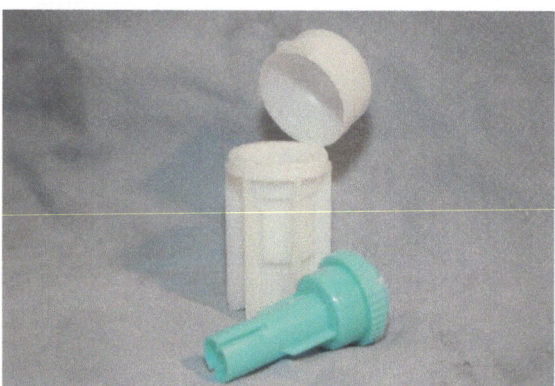
Figure 71: Fecalizer cup

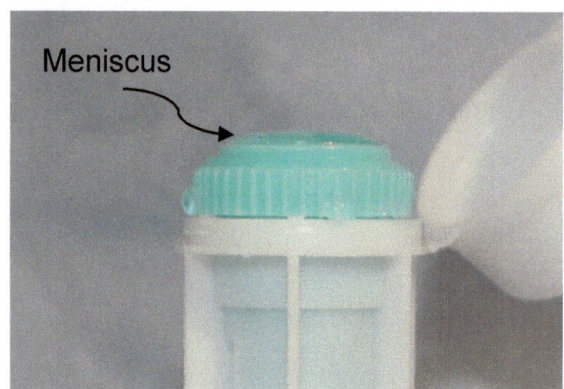
Meniscus
Figure 72: Fluid meniscus on top of fecalizer

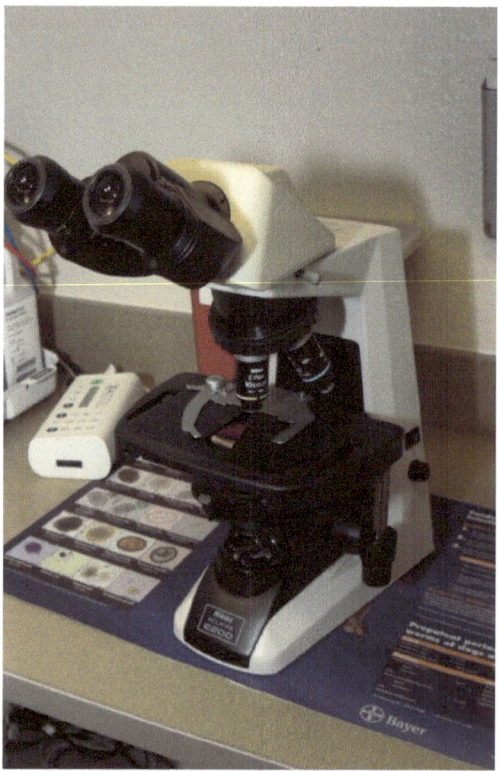
Figure 73: Binocular microscope

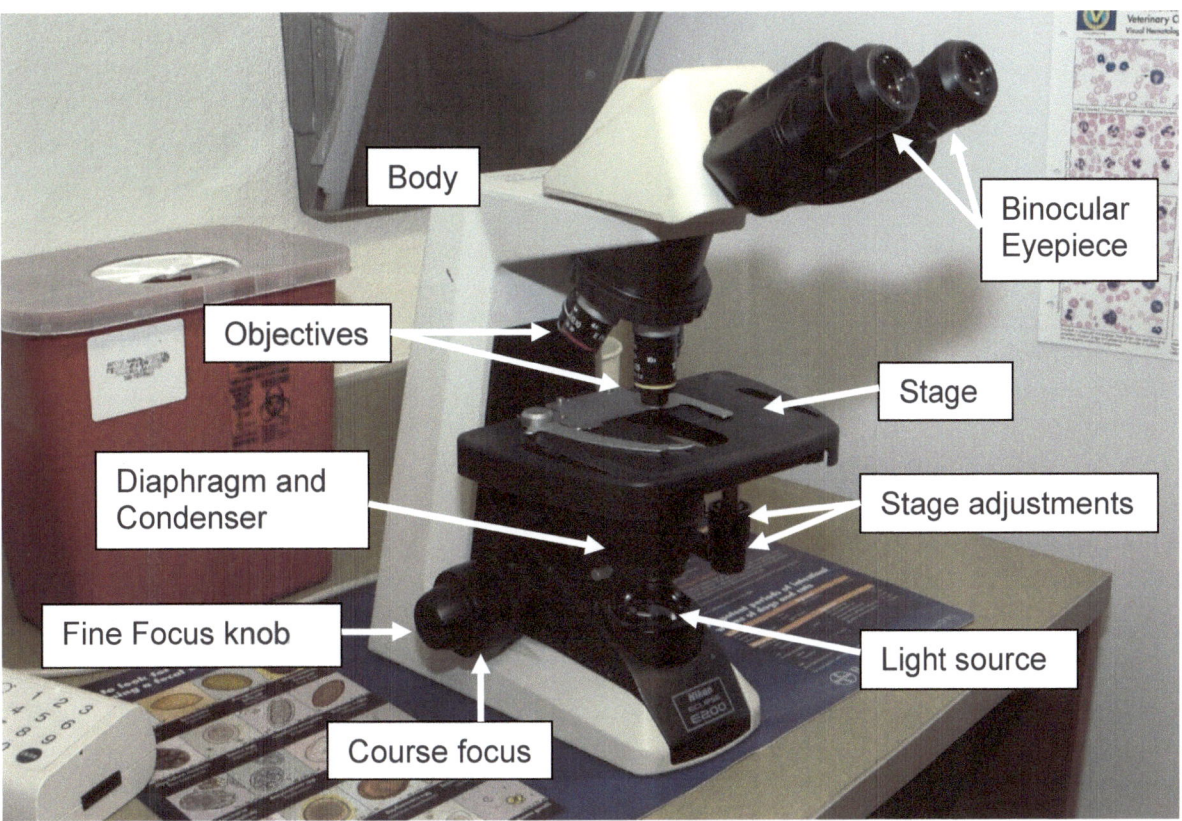

Figure 74: Components of the microscope

The most common endoparasites of companion animals are the roundworm and tapeworm; the roundworm looks like a piece of spaghetti, and the tapeworm looks like pieces of rice.

Diagnostic Imaging

Diagnostic imaging is a valuable tool in veterinary medicine. Radiologic imaging is the most common form of imaging used in veterinary practices, as it is informative and is relatively cost effective. Radiologic images, or x-rays, enable veterinarians to see the internal structures of the body in a minimally invasive way; the only requirement is for the patient to hold still.

X-rays

The fundamental component of a radiographic image is the x-ray. X-rays are high-energy electromagnetic waves, which can effectively pass through living tissues like skin and organs. The wavelength is above the visible spectrum, and, therefore, is invisible to the naked eye. X-rays, first discovered by Conrad Roentgen, are a form of ionizing radiation that has the ability to break chemical bonds and mutate DNA in the body. Other effects include erythema of the skin, eye damage, and for this reason, x-ray radiation safety is an important consideration for the veterinary team. Several laws and safety practices have been enacted to ensure the safety of the veterinary team when working with, or around, x-rays. These laws and recommendations ensure that veterinary professionals limit the damaging effects of x-ray radiation and reduce their occupational exposure over the course of their careers.

- By law, individuals under 18 years of age cannot take x-rays in a veterinary practice.
- By law, pregnant individuals cannot take x-rays in a veterinary practice.
- Protective attire should be worn to limit exposure to x-ray radiation.
- Individuals should always avoid placing any part of their body in the primary x-ray beam.

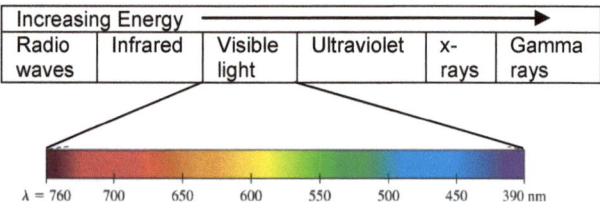

Figure 75: The electromagnetic spectrum

Other ways to reduce one's occupational exposure to x-ray radiation, includes reducing the number of x-ray exposures and the duration of each exposure. Additionally, increasing the distance from the primary beam and using proper shielding equipment will reduce one's exposure.

The Three Amigos

Occupational exposure of x-ray radiation can be significantly reduced if one remembers the Three Amigos of radiation safety:

- Time
- Distance
- Shielding

X-ray machines are like cameras; they utilize the same fundamental principles. The longer the exposure setting on the camera, the more light is allowed to expose the film. The same holds true for radiographic images. By reducing the time of exposure, radiation exposure is reduced. Retaking a radiograph because of improper technique or poor positioning can increase one's exposure to radiation. These retakes increase the time one is potentially exposed to radiation.

X-rays easily penetrate through tissue; however, they don't travel very far. By increasing one's distance from the x-ray beam, the potential exposure can be significantly reduced. The inverse square law states that as the distance from the x-ray beam doubles, the x-ray beam intensity decreases by a factor of four. For example, if an x-ray beam produces one rem of radiation at one foot, at two feet, it would produce one quarter of that, or 0.25rem. A rem, or Roentgen equivalent man, is a quantitative unit of radiation exposure or dose equivalent. Exposure to natural background radiation in one year produces less than 0.1rem, whereas a dose of more than 1000rem is usually fatal.

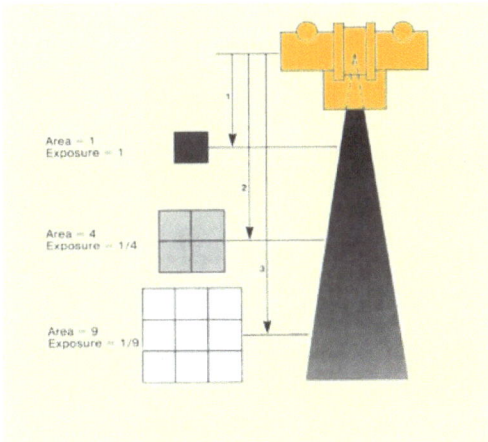

Figure 76: Inverse square law

X-rays are attenuated by concrete and lead. Shielding involves the use of these materials to protect veterinary personnel from radiation exposure. The most common forms of personal shielding attire are the lead apron, gloves and thyroid protector. The attire is heavy and bulky, but allows enough flexibility to be functional while holding animals for radiographs. The protective clothing is designed to protect especially sensitive body parts including the thyroid glands, reproductive organs and extremities. Even though protective clothing prevents the penetration of x-ray radiation, care should be taken to avoid exposure to the primary beam even while wearing this attire. Leaded glass and moveable wall barriers are sometimes utilized in the radiology suite. These allow veterinary staff to safely operate radiographic equipment.

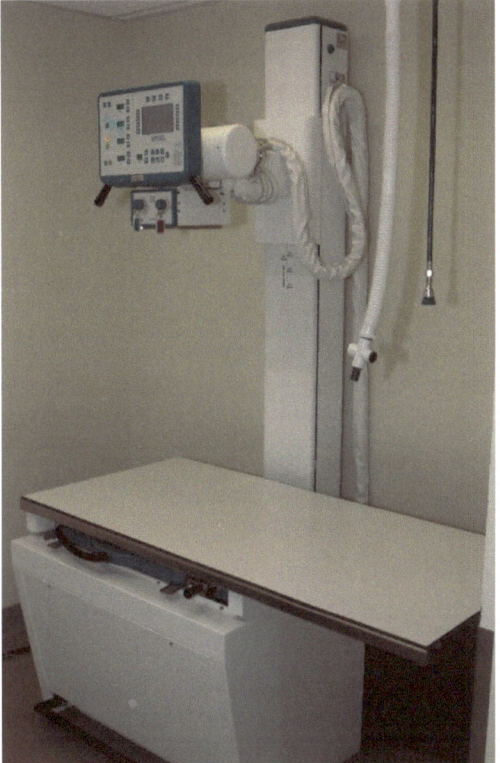

Figure 77: Small animal x-ray machine

Radiology Terms

mAs or Milliamperage-second is a quantitative exposure factor. This setting on the x-ray machine determines the amount of x-rays being sent out of the machine and the length of exposure. The mAs is often determined by the region of the patient being radiographed. The mAs gives an x-ray contrast.

KVP or Kilovoltage peak is a qualitative exposure factor. This setting on the x-ray machine determines the quality of the x-rays being sent through the patient. This setting is usually determined by the patient's thickness. The KVP gives an x-ray its shades of gray.

Not all x-rays penetrate through the patient; some are deflected. *Scatter* is the deflection of x-rays off the patient, and attributes to one's occupational exposure to x-ray radiation. Protective attire (shielding) and beam collimation reduces the effect of scatter.

Grids are used in some cases to reduce the blurring of x-ray images that scatter creates. Grids are plates that only allow x-rays at right angles through; this eliminates deflected x-rays from reaching the film or digital plate.

Focal film distance is the distance from the x-ray head to the film or digital panel. The focal film distance is usually fixed, but many x-ray machines have the ability to adjust this distance.

Analog film has traditionally been used for x-ray imagery. Just as a film camera, x-ray film uses plain film to generate an image. X-ray film is stored in a light proof container called a cassette, and once exposed, is developed by the use of a chemical film processor. Both the film and cassettes come in a variety of film and screen types to enable high-resolution images. Analog film systems are being replaced by digital technology, partially because of the expense of x-ray film and chemicals, and their waste. Digital technology, just as a digital camera, captures x-ray images on a phosphor plate. Images are processed by a computer instead of a chemical processor. Digital images can be easily manipulated, stored, and shared at the click of a button. Digital technology utilizes the same x-rays as traditional analog film.

Patient information must be noted on every piece of x-ray film. Digital systems embed patient information at the time the radiograph is taken. Analog film requires an imprint to be placed directly on the film. An x-ray imprinter is used to expose patient information onto the film. The imprinter is located in the darkroom, and used prior to developing the film.

Analog x-ray film must be handled and processed in a darkroom.

Patient Positioning

An x-ray produces a two dimensional image. In order to see a 'complete picture' of a patient, a second view is generally taken. This view, usually perpendicular (90 degrees) to the first, enables the veterinarian to essentially obtain a 3rd dimension.

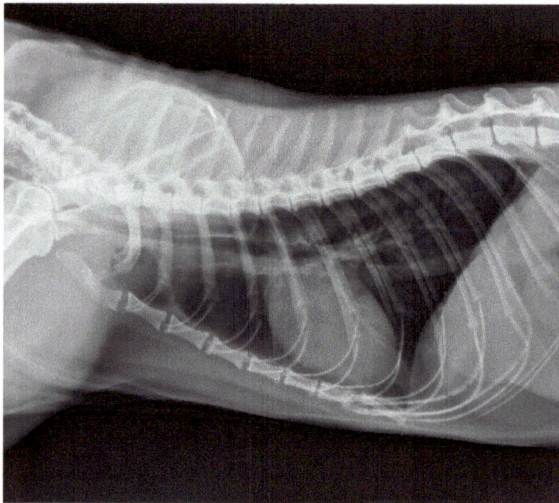

Figure 78: Right lateral view

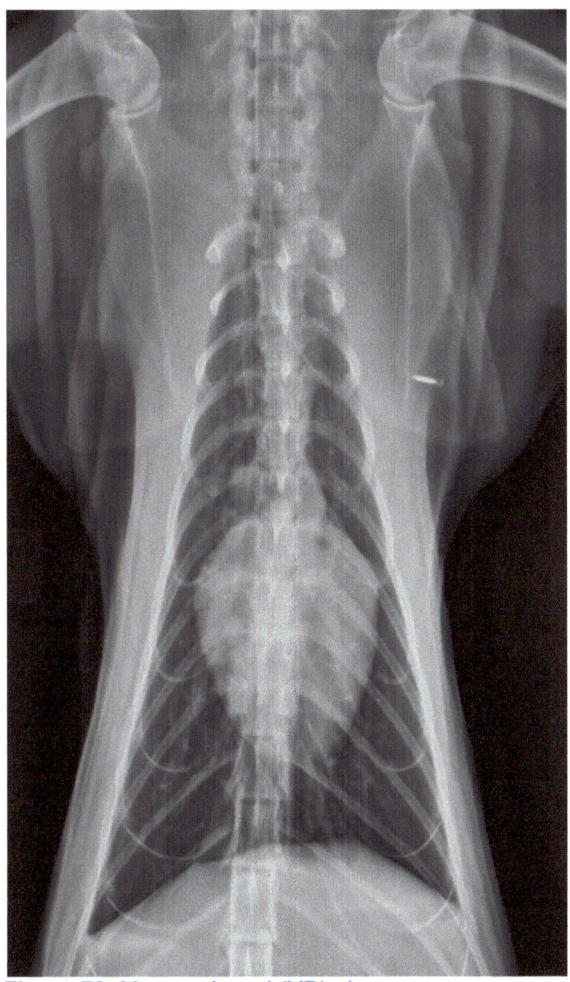

Figure 79: Ventro-dorsal (VD) view

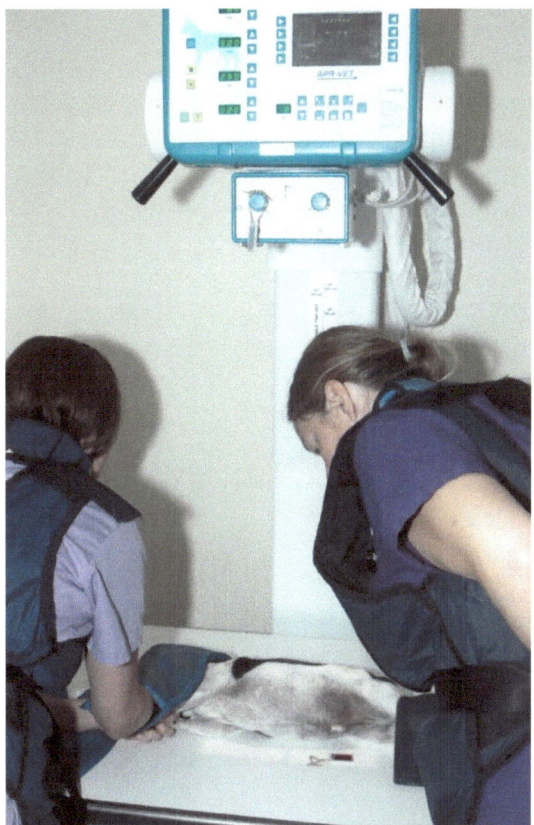

Figure 80: Patient placed in right lateral recumbency for radiograph

When taking chest radiographs, for example, the patient is often placed in right lateral recumbency (right side of the body on the x-ray table) for the first image, followed by a ventral/dorsal position (back on the x-ray table with feet pointing up) for the second image. The patient's positioning is generally based on the region being radiographed. Positioning aids such as foam pads, rope and tape may be used to optimize patient position for radiographs. Proper positioning will reduce the number of retakes necessary, and reduce one's occupational exposure to x-ray radiation.

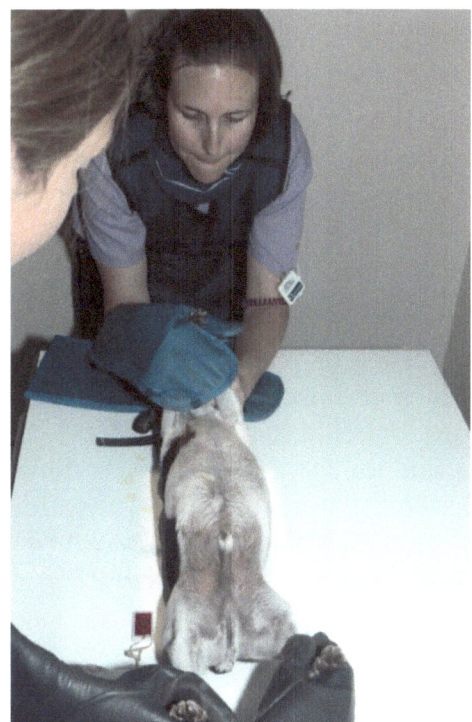

Figure 81: Dog positioned for ventro-dorsal (VD) radiograph

Appearance of Radiographs

Radiographic images lack color; images are black and white with shades of gray. A radiograph will appear black after being exposed to x-ray radiation. Bones attenuate most x-rays and prevent x-rays from reaching the film; the result is white, underexposed areas on the film.

Metal, such as lead, attenuates all x-rays and produces the whitest areas. Likewise, a patient's air-filled lungs attenuate few x-rays, and therefore appear nearly black on the film. Organs and muscles are somewhere between bone and lung, producing shades of gray on the film.

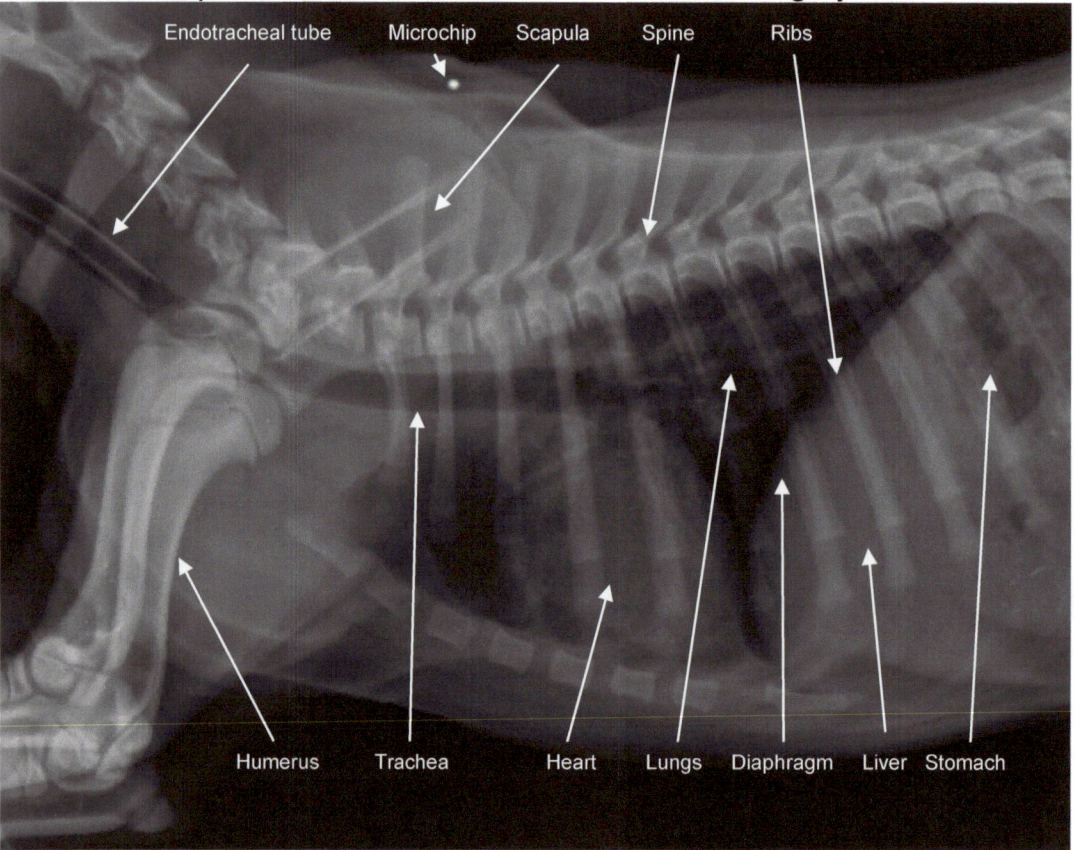

Figure 82: Right lateral thorax radiograph

Technique Chart

A technique chart is used to optimize the black, white and grays of a radiographic image. Technique is based on the region being radiographed as well as patient thickness. As patient increases, more x-ray energy is needed to penetrate it. Technique charts can be variable in design, but functionally provide the necessary information to take a diagnostic radiograph.

The steps to interpreting a technique chart include the following:

1. Determine the region being radiographed
2. Locate the proper mAs based on that region
3. Determine the patient thickness, in centimeters, of the region being radiographed
4. Locate the proper KVP based on the patient thickness

Once the mAs and KVP have been determined, the patient can be positioned for the radiographs.

Remember to take measurements for both views, as these thicknesses may be significantly different.

Region	mAs	Patient thickness(cm)→	4	5	6	7	8	9	10
Thorax	1.0	KVP→	70	72	74	76	78	80	82
Abdomen	2.0		66	68	70	72	74	76	78
Spine/skull	5.0		58	60	62	66	68	70	72
Extremities	6.0		56	58	60	62	64	66	68

Table 16: Radiographic Technique Chart

Other Modalities

Advances in computer technology have greatly expanded the use of x-rays. Analog radiographic film has given way to digital images; film processors are being replaced with computers. Radiology is now used to diagnose and treat disease. Several x-ray modalities are now being used in veterinary medicine.

Computed Axial Tomography, or the CAT scan, uses x-rays to produce image slices of the body. These slices can be manipulated by a computer to produce a 3 dimensional image.

Scintigraphy is used to identify and diagnose cancers in the body. Unlike x-ray technology, radioisotopes are placed in the animal, and the emitted radiation is captured by the scintigraphy detectors.

Fluoroscopy, or real time x-rays, are used for cardiac surgery and procedures requiring 'x-ray guidance'.

> **KVP increases by two for every cm increase in patient's thickness.**

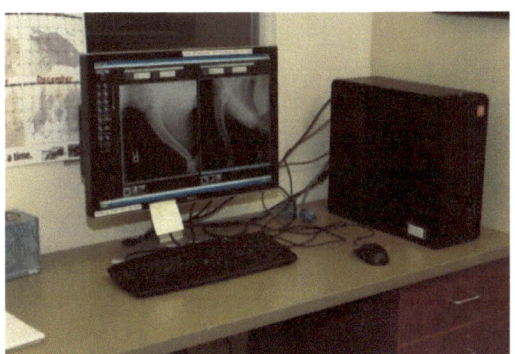

Figure 83: Computer based radiographic images

Surgery

Surgery, once considered the art of working with one's hands, is now known as a capable scientific discipline, where disease and ailments are treated by manipulation of bodily structures. Early surgical procedures included bloodletting, and trepanation, or drilling a pressure-relieving hole into the head. This procedure was designed to treat health problems associated with intracranial pressure and other diseases. Advances in hemostasis, pain management and infection, allowed the art of surgery to become a modern science. Modern surgery is not limited to cutting into the patient and may include other procedures requiring anesthesia.

Types of surgery

Elective surgeries are those that are generally scheduled in advance. These are surgical procedures that have been decided on and planned. Spays, neuters, declawing, lumpectomies and dental prophylaxis are examples of elective procedures.

Surgical term	Common term
Ovariohysterectomy	Spay
Orchiectomy	Neuter
Onychectomy	Declaw

Table 17: Common Elective Surgical Terms

Some male dogs and cats may lack one or both testicles in the scrotum. This requires more involved surgical means to perform a neuter. The condition called anorchid, meaning 'without flower', and cryptorchid meaning 'hidden flower' refers to this condition. In some cases, exploratory laparotomy is needed to find the undescended testicle. A neuter completely removes the testicles; whereas, a vasectomy simply interrupts the connection between the testicles and the reproductive tract, leaving the testicles intact.

Non-elective surgeries are non-scheduled or emergency procedures. Examples include cesarean sections, exploratory laparotomies, fracture and wound repair and other traumatic injuries. Because of the 'emergency' nature of the procedure, pre anesthetic blood testing and fasting may have not been accomplished. Additionally, these patients may have trauma or injuries that make them a high anesthetic risk.

Surgical term	Common term
Cesarean section	C-section or surgical birth
Exploratory laparotomy	Surgical exploration of the abdomen
Cystotomy	Surgery of the bladder
Herniorrhaphy	Hernia repair
Tarsorrhaphy	Surgical closure of the eyelids
Urethrostomy	Surgical opening of the urethra

Table 18: Non-elective Surgical Terms

Pre-operative Considerations

Several considerations must be made prior to any surgical procedure. Patient age should initially be considered. The older the patient, the weaker and more compromised the organ systems may be. This may also cause prolonged recoveries. Anesthesia and surgery can be taxing on the body; patient health is important to assess prior to surgery. Most anesthetics are metabolized by the liver and kidneys, and therefore should be evaluated. A pre-operative physical exam and blood work should be standard practice for most animals. In addition, a detailed history of seizure disorders and drug allergies should be obtained, as some anesthetics and sedatives lower the seizure threshold in animals.

Prior to any anesthetic procedure, animals should have all food and water withheld. This is to ensure that no food or water could be regurgitated and aspirated into the lungs during or while recovering from anesthesia. This is often referred to as 'fasting', and may be abbreviated NPO, meaning no per os. For carnivores like dogs and cats that have a relatively short GI transit time, a 12-hour fasting is generally sufficient to ensure an empty stomach. Some species, such as herbivores, require additional fasting time. Other species, such as small birds may require a much shorter fasting time.

Prior to surgery, the patient is usually given a pre-anesthetic medication, followed by a general anesthetic. General anesthesia facilitates patient unconsciousness and enables pain free surgery. Once under anesthesia, the patient can be prepared for the surgical procedure.

> **NPO means no per os, or no food and water prior to a surgical procedure.**

Surgical Preparation-Patient
The initial process of surgical preparation involves several steps:
- Patient positioning
- Clipping of surgical site
- Emptying bladder if needed
- Aseptically cleaning surgical site

Patient positioning is based on the type of surgery being performed. For most elective procedures, the patient is placed on their back, with feet secured to the surgical table. The patient should be secured sufficiently enough so not to shift during surgery.

Clipping of the surgical site requires the use of a hair clipper; a number 40 clipper blade allows for complete hair removal. Caution should be used, however, to prevent clipper burn. Large margins should be clipped around the surgical site to prevent the possibility of hair getting into the surgical area. A water-based lubricant such as KY can be placed in open wounds to prevent clipped hair from getting into the wound.

Emptying the bladder may be beneficial for abdominal surgeries. The bladder, a large fluid filled sac, can obscure other structures in the abdomen, if not emptied. Caution should be used when emptying the bladder, as possible rupture can occur if done improperly.

Aseptically cleaning of the surgical site is the most important pre-surgical step. A common technique is called the 'triple prep'. This process involves the use of antiseptic soap and isopropyl alcohol; soap and alcohol are alternated to provide an aseptic surgical field. The steps are as follows:

1. Using an antiseptic soap soaked gauze sponge, apply and scrub the surgical site from the center to the outside edges.
2. Follow step one with an alcohol soaked gauze sponge, cleaning from the center of the surgical site to the outside edges.
3. Repeat steps 1 and 2 at least 3 times. After the 3rd time, if the gauze sponge is still soiled, continue the steps until it is clean.
4. Place an antiseptic solution such as chlorhexadine or betadine on the surgical field following the 'triple prep'.

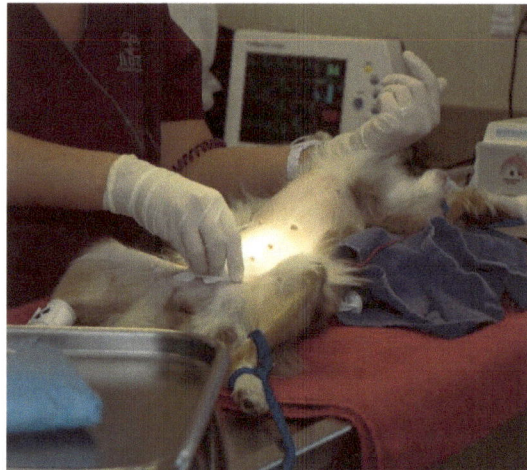

Figure 84: Surgical site preparation

Increased soap contact time is always better when cleaning.

Surgical Preparation-Surgical Staff

The surgeon and surgical support staff must also be 'prepped' for surgery. Surgical caps and masks are worn by the surgical team to reduce contamination of the surgical field. Additionally, surgical gowns and gloves are worn to ensure a sterile setting for the patient; any contamination could lead to infection for the patient.

The steps for staff prep are as follows:

1. Put on surgical cap and mask. These items are not sterile so do not touch them while in surgery.
2. Aseptically scrub hands; increased soap contact time is always more effective.
3. Rinse with hands higher than elbows to prevent dirty soap from running down to hands.
4. Dry hands with a sterile towel
5. Carefully, put on surgical gown without contaminating outside surface.
6. Carefully, put on surgical gloves.

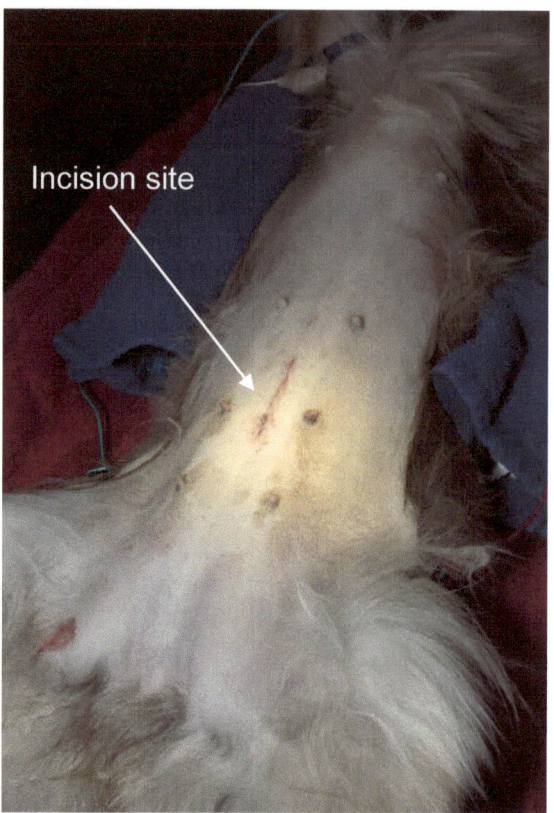

Incision site

Figure 85: Post-surgical spay incision

Surgical Preparation-Equipment

Surgical equipment must be properly sterilized and wrapped to prevent contamination. Wrapping and sterilizing packs, gowns, drapes and instruments are important tasks of the veterinary assistant. Understanding sterile fields, presentation, cleaning, and instrument identification is essential. Steam and gas sterilization are the most common ways surgical equipment are sterilized, and therefore, the use of this equipment must be understood.

Gowns may be disposable or reusable. Reusable gowns are generally made of a durable cloth material that is safe for machine washing. Reusable gowns are wrapped so the outside of the gown gets rolled inward toward the center of the gown. This ensures that the outside of the gown is sterile when put on. Gowns are folded and wrapped with muslin drape material; a steam sterilization indicator should be placed inside so proper sterilization can easily be determined. The steam indicator changes color when exposed to steam sterilization. Reusable drapes are folded and sterilized in the same manner as gowns. They can be wrapped in muslin, or placed into a seal pouch for sterilization. Seal pouches have indicators that change color when exposed to steam or gas sterilization. Instruments can be wrapped individually in seal pouches, or as a group in a 'pack'. A pack contains instruments commonly used for specific surgical procedures such as spays and neuters. A 'spay pack' will contain instruments necessary to perform a surgical spay. Packs are wrapped in muslin drapes and have a steam indicator placed inside. Some packs may include drapes and gauze.

Autoclave tape is used to determine whether a wrapped gown, drape, or pack has been autoclaved. Autoclave tape looks like masking tape, but black lines are produced when exposed to steam sterilization. The steam indicator on the inside confirms the penetration of steam into the center of the gown.

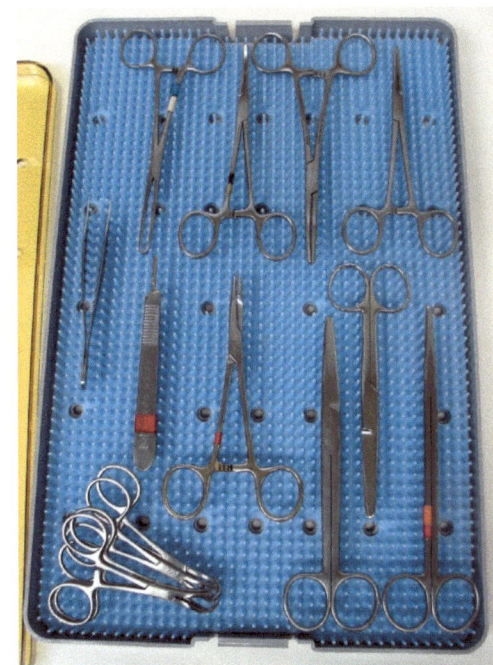
Figure 87: Instrument Pack

Autoclave tape appears striped when exposed to steam sterilization.

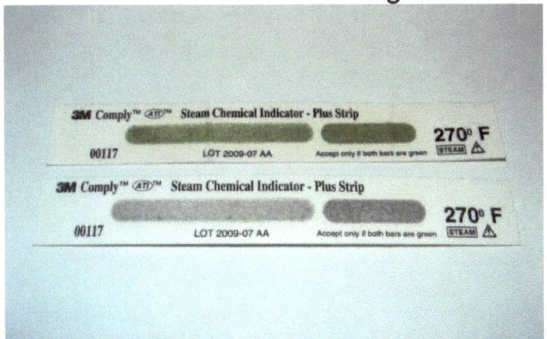
Figure 86: Indicator strip showing color change to green (top) after being exposed to steam sterilization

Wrapping an Instrument Pack

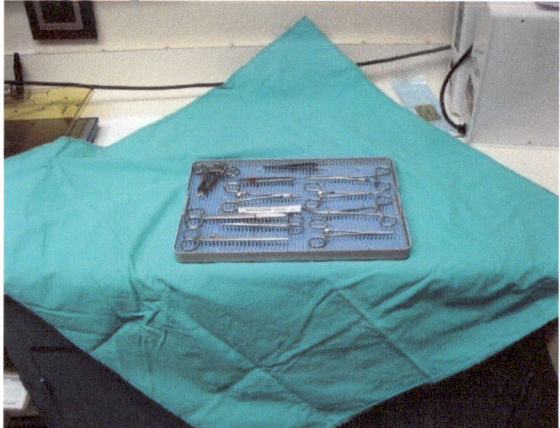

Step 1: Place pack in center of wrap.

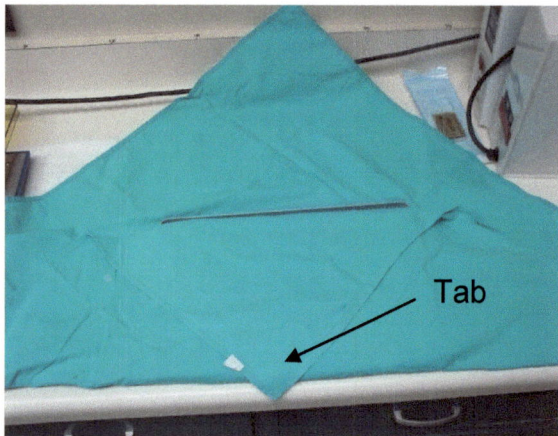

Step 2: Fold one edge of wrap over pack leaving a tab.

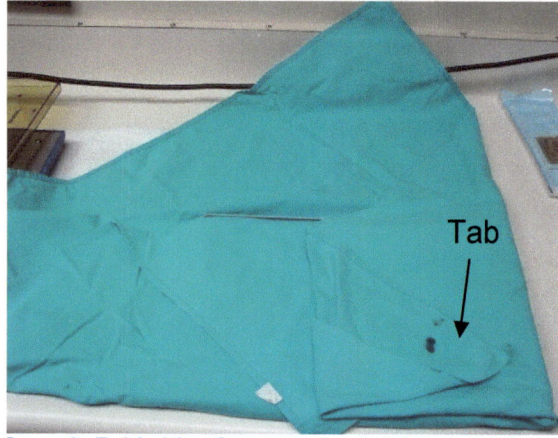

Step 3: Fold side of wrap over pack leaving tab.

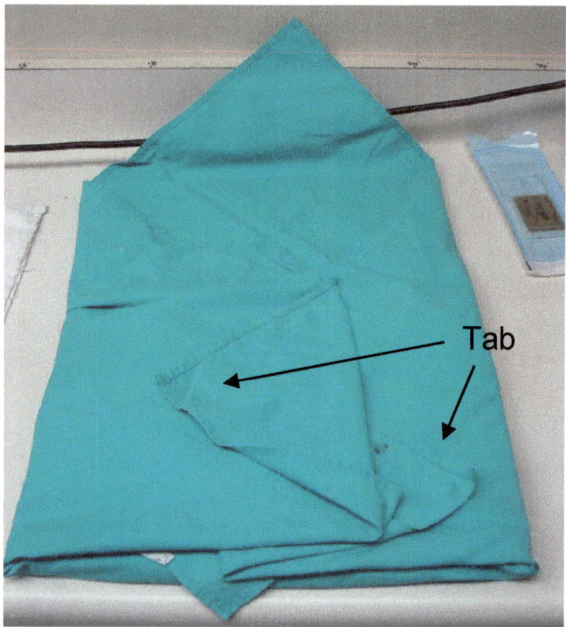

Step 4: Fold other side of wrap over pack leaving tab.

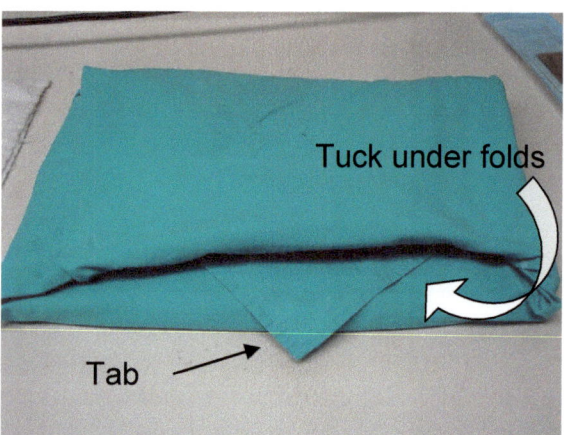

Step 5: Fold top of wrap over pack and tuck under other folds leaving a tab.

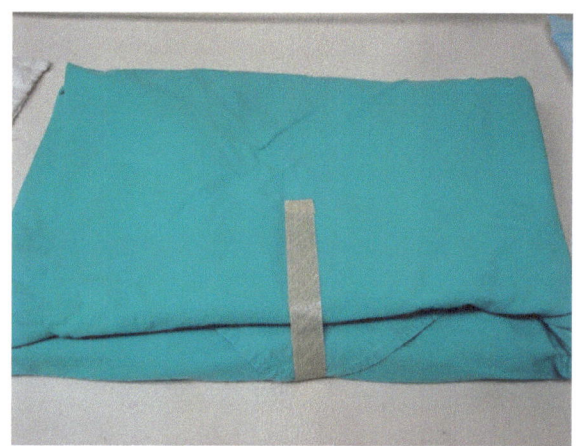

Step 6: Secure pack with autoclave tape, and label contents of pack.

Gowns, drapes, instruments and packs are opened in the opposite order that they are packed. When opening a pack, for example, it should be assumed that the contents are sterile, and no contact should be made with the interior except by the surgeon. In order to maintain a sterile field, avoid moving one's hands over the opened instrument packs or the patient after surgical preparation. Instruments are usually placed on a surgical table and draped in such a way to provide a sterile platform from which the surgeon can work.

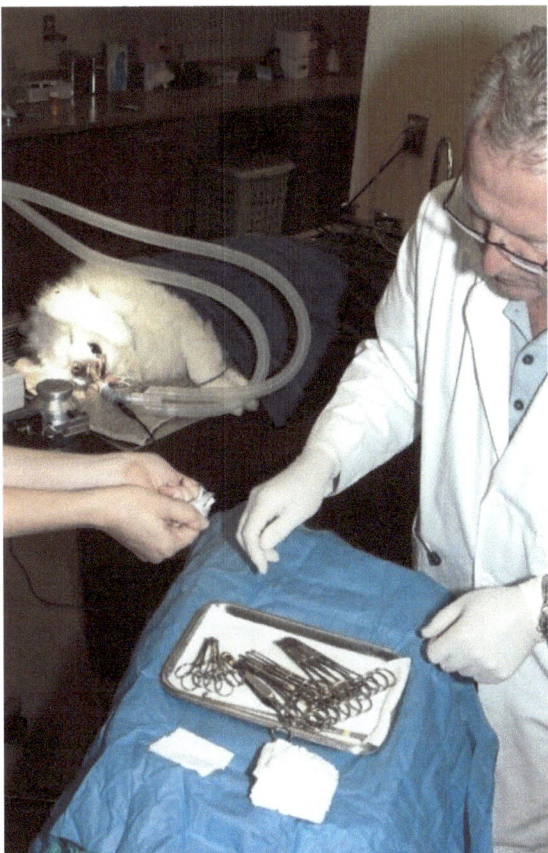
Figure 89: Surgeon and sterile instruments. Note assistant (left) giving surgeon surgical blade without disturbing sterile field.

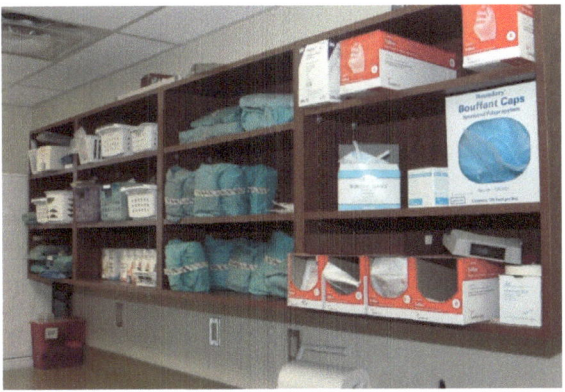
Figure 88: Sterile surgical supplies

After surgery, soiled, reusable gowns and drapes can be placed in the washing machine. Linens can be soaked in an enzymatic cleaner prior to washing, so blood and biological material can be effectively removed. If not removed, blood can leave stains on linens. Instruments must be thoroughly cleaned prior to being sterilized. Cleaning brushes and antiseptic soap can be used to clean all surfaces of instruments. Following the initial cleaning, instruments can be placed in an ultrasonic cleaner to remove any hard to reach debris. Instruments should be placed in 'instrument milk', a lubricant, to ensure proper functioning and longevity of expensive surgical equipment.

Surgical Instruments

Surgical instruments are an essential part of any surgical procedure. They are expensive, high quality, precision tools used to perform a multitude of tasks. The basic components of a surgical instrument include:

- Tip
- Jaws
- Box lock
- Shank
- Ratchet
- Ring handle

Commonly used surgical instruments include the following:

Needle holders are used to hold a needle and assist with suturing wounds and incisions. Some needle holders have a cutting surface for cutting suture material.

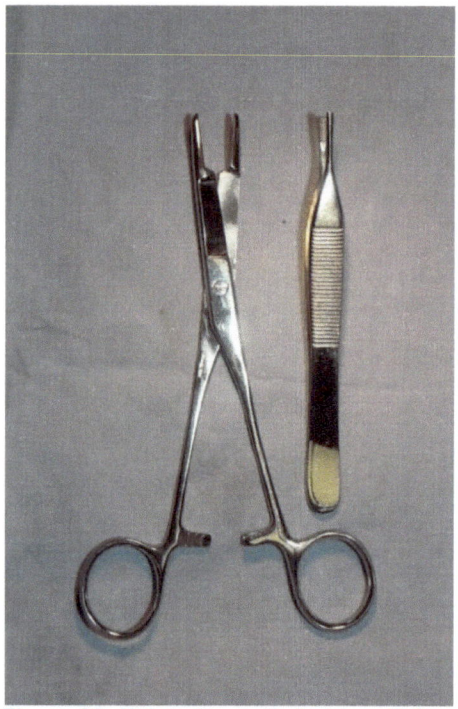

Figure 90: Halstedt needle holders (left) and thumb forcep

Scalpel handles are used to make incisions. One of many blade types can be attached to the scalpel handle depending on the type of surgery or incision needed. Some scalpel blades are curved, pointed, or blunted.

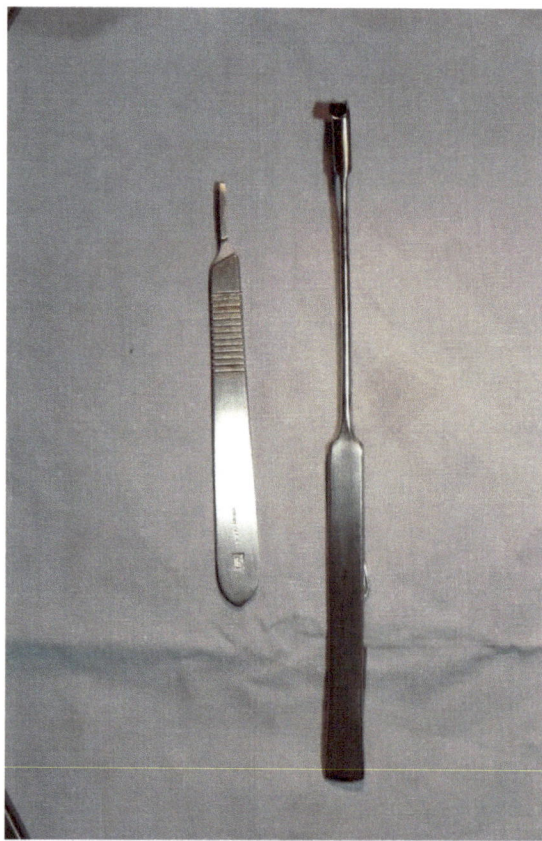

Figure 91: Scalpel handle (left) and spay hook

Scissors come in a variety of shapes, sizes and functions. Some are designed for cutting suture and tough materials like muscle, while others are designed for delicate cutting and dissection. Three common types used in veterinary medicine include the operating, mayo dissecting and metzenbaum dissecting scissors.

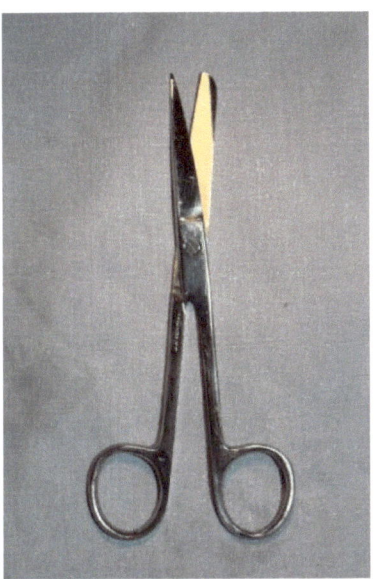

Figure 92: Sharp blunt scissors

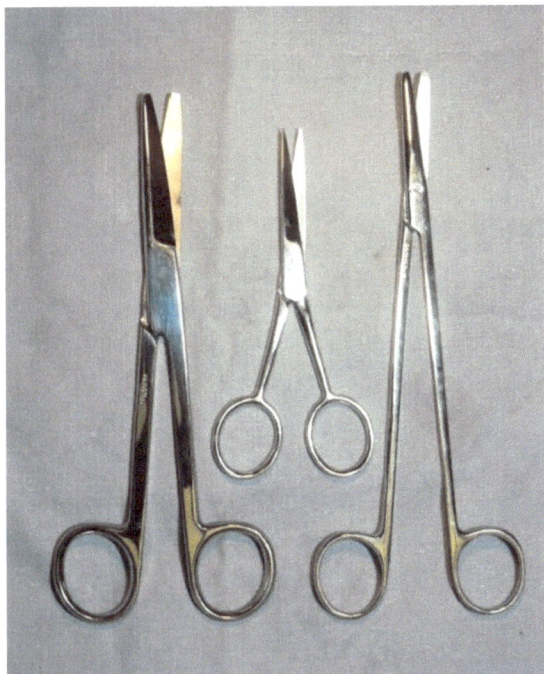

Figure 93: Mayo (left), dissecting (center) and metzenbaum scissors (right)

Thumb Forceps are used to grab and manipulate tissue. Also called 'pick-ups', thumb forceps are commonly used in conjunction with needle holders to assist with placement of sutures in the patient. Thumb forceps have a variety of teeth types, including the rat tooth or serrated tip, smooth tip and cross-hatched dressing tip.

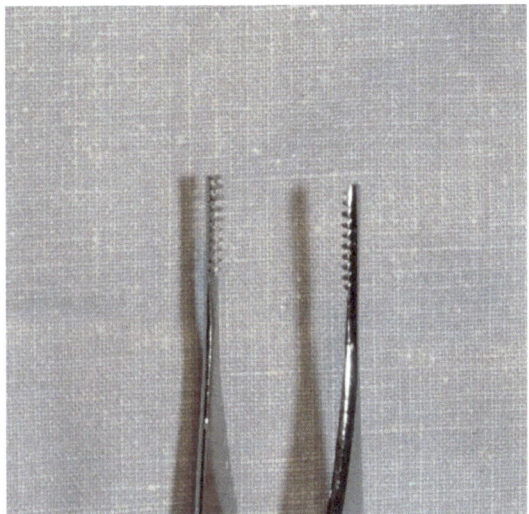

Figure 94: Serrated tips of a thumb forcep

Tissue forceps are similar to thumb forceps in function, but can be locked; this enables tissues and blood vessels to be grasped and clamped. Common types tissue forceps include the 'hemostats' such as the *Halsted mosquito forceps* and the larger *Kelly* and *Crile* forceps. *Rochester-Carmalts* are used for clamping very large vessels such as those found in the uterus during a spay surgery. *Allis tissue forceps* are designed as a tissue clamping retractor.

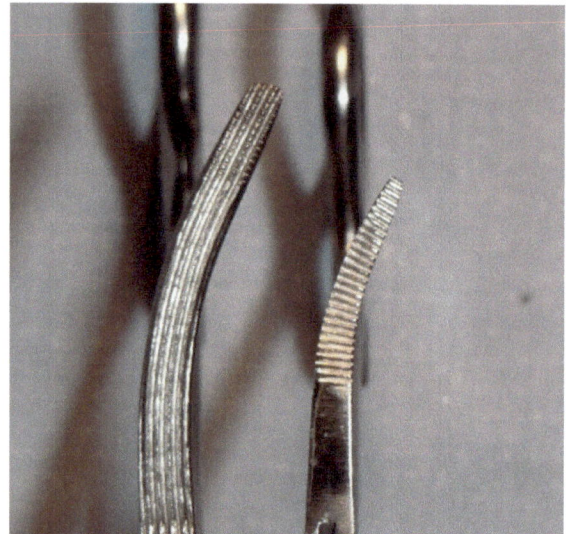

Figure 95: Differences in serration direction of the carmalt (left) and mosquito hemostat

Backhaus towel clamps are used to secure surgical drapes to the patient. This ensures that the position of the drape remains constant, and the sterile field is not compromised.

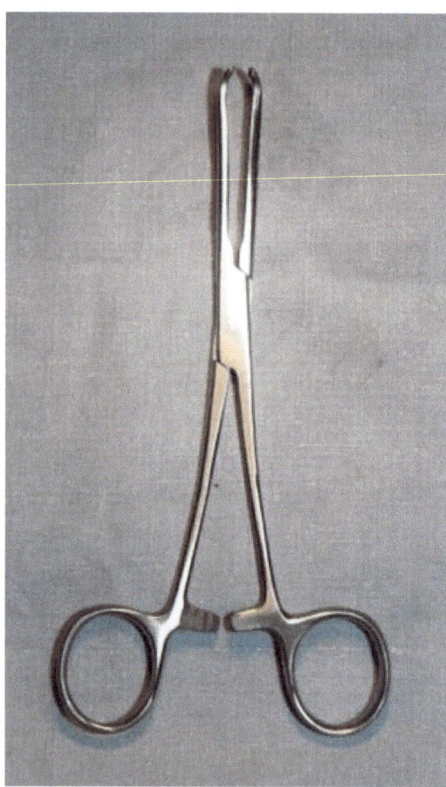

Figure 96: Allis retractor

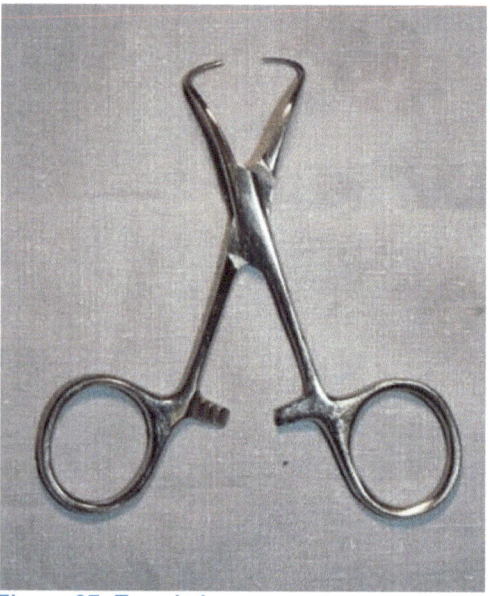

Figure 97: Towel clamp

Snook ovariohysterectomy hooks are used to pull the uterine horns through the incision area of a spay surgery. This enables the surgeon to create a relatively small incision.

Other specialized instruments may be needed based on the surgery type and complexity. These may include:
Hand held retractors
- Senn
- Army-Navy
- Murphy

Self-retaining retractors
- Balfour
- Gelpi
- Weitlaner

Orthopedic instruments
- Bone holding forceps
- Periosteal elevators
- Curettes
- Chisels
- Gigli wire
- Bone pins/wires

Suction
- Frazier
- Poole

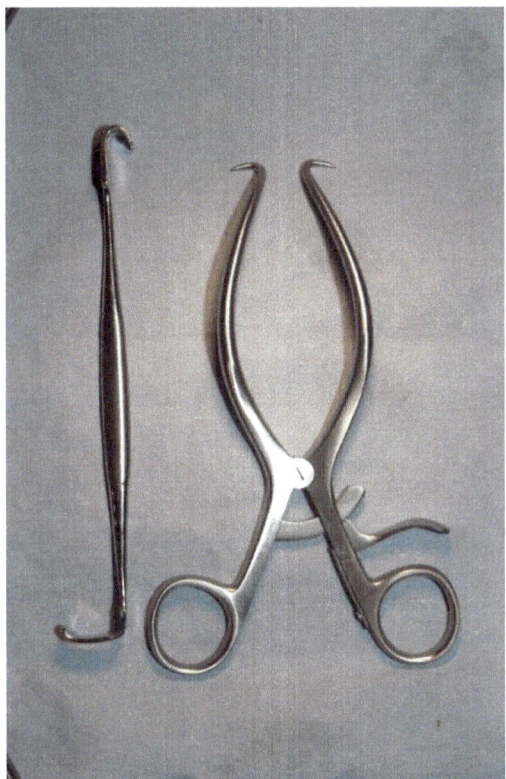

Figure 98: Senn (left) and Gelpi retractors

Suture material is primarily used for closing surgical incisions, but can also be used for skin retraction and ligation of blood vessels. Suture material comes in a variety of sizes and materials, and in some cases, comes with a needle already attached to it. Bulk suture material comes in sterile spools and requires the attachment of a needle; this system is designed to reduce the waste caused by pre-cut suture packs, as the surgeon only takes the amount of suture that is needed. Threading the needle is the main challenge with this system; a supply of needles must be available. Swaged-on suture and needle combinations are popular because of their convenience. Needles are already attached to the suture material, and the attachment point is seamless so the needle and suture move through the tissue more easily. Suture waste is a problem, as the 'packs' have a pre-measured amount of suture present, and these packs are more expensive.

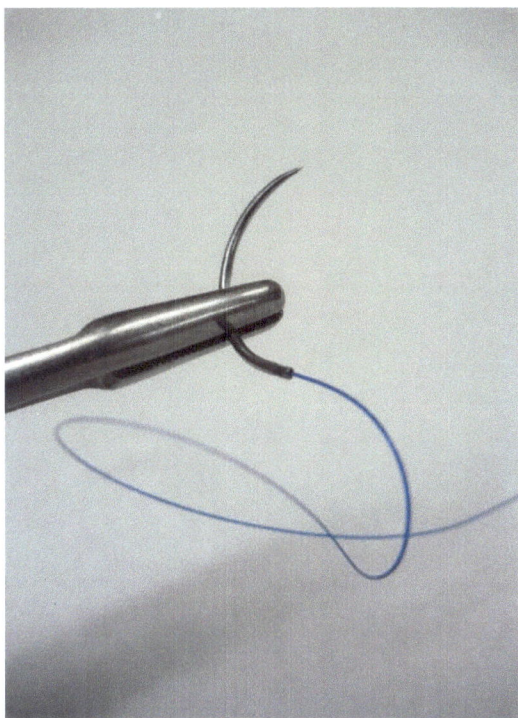

Figure 99: Swagged-on needle and suture

Suture material types include the following:

- Absorbable
- Non-absorbable
- Monofilament
- Multifilament or braided

Selection of suture material is based on whether the surgeon wants the material to be absorbed by the body (absorbable) or maintained for long periods (non-absorbable). Monofilament suture tends to be less reactive and inflammatory than braided; however, it tends to be more difficult with which to work.

Suture material comes in a variety of thicknesses; thicker suture is designed for thicker tissues and closures, and increased tensile strength. Suture comes in sizes ranging from #7USP (0.9mm), to #11-0 (0.01mm). Common suture diameters used in veterinary practices range from #0 to #4-0.

Absorbable suture material is dissolved by the patient, and non-absorbable suture material does not dissolve and is removed at some point after the surgery.

Suture Type	Absorbable	Non-absorbable	Monofilament	Multifilament
Chromic gut	•			•
Vicryl	•			•
PDS	•		•	
Monocryl	•		•	
Dexon	•			•
Maxon	•		•	
Prolene		•	•	
Vetafil		•		•

Table 19: Common suture types

Needles are separated into 2 types, cutting and taper tips. Needles may also be curved or straight. Curved needles are common because of the ease in which they can be used in small areas. Needle diameters vary, but are generally similar to the suture diameter being used.

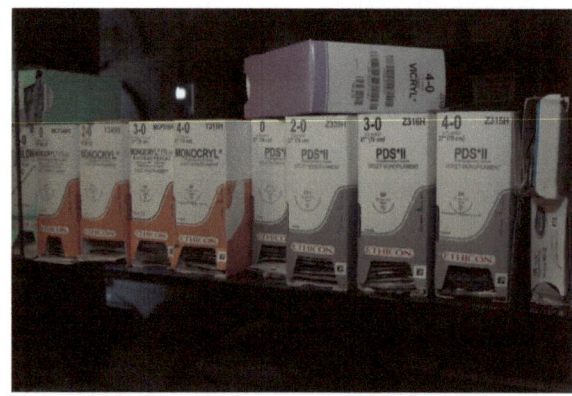

Figure 100: Assorted suture material

Cutting needles have a triangular shape and are designed for cutting through tissues. The triangular edges are sharp and can cut through tough skin easily. These needles are not designed for delicate tissues and organs due to the traumatic means in which they cut through the tissue.

Taper needles are smooth with a sharp pointed tip. These needles are designed for suturing organs and delicate tissues.

Anesthesia

Anesthesia can be defined as loss of bodily sensation with or without unconsciousness. Anesthetics are designed to provide analgesia or pain relief, amnesia and immobilization. Anesthetics are used to facilitate surgical procedures. Types of anesthesia used in veterinary medicine include local, regional and general anesthesia.

Local anesthesia is used to anesthetize local or specific areas. Examples include: wound and mole removal. *Regional blocks* are designed to anesthetize larger regions. They include epidural, spinal and ring blocks. *General anesthesia* is the most common type and is designed to anesthetize the whole patient. This is the preferred method of anesthetic use because it completely immobilizes the patient, and prevents possible injury.

Anesthetics can be delivered to the patient into the muscle (IM), subcutaneously (SQ), intravenously (IV), or by gas inhalation. In some cases, pre-anesthetic sedatives are used to ease the anesthetic induction process. These sedative combinations are also designed to increase and stabilize the patient's heart rate, as well as reduce salivation and GI motility; all important considerations for anesthesia. Some anesthetics, also known as agonists, can be 'reversed' or antagonized with drugs designed to negate their effects. For example, the effects of medetomidine, a potent α2 (alpha 2) sedative, can be completely reversed with the drug, atipamezole. Benefits include a more rapid recovery,

and the ability to lighten the level of anesthesia easily.

The effects of anesthetic drugs on the body may include changes in thermoregulation, cardiac output and respiration. Although, it is the role for the anesthetist to monitor these changes, it is important for all veterinary support personnel to understand and alert the surgeon of changes in these physiological parameters.

Type	Route	Examples
Local	IM, SQ	Lidocaine Bupivicaine
Chemical	IM, IV IV IM IM IM IV	Ketamine Diazepam Midazolam Medetomidine Butorphanol Propofol
Gas	Inhalant	Halothane Isoflurane Sevoflurane Desflurane

Table 20: Common Anesthetic drugs and routes

The anesthetic induction process begins with the administration of a chemical anesthetic. In small animal practices, this is usually delivered IV. The drug or 'cocktail' used generally renders the patient unconscious in a matter of seconds. An airway is then established with the use of an endotracheal tube. This tube, when connected to the anesthetic machine, will allow the patient to breathe without the risk of occlusion or aspiration into the trachea. Intubation is facilitated by the use of a laryngoscope. This hand-held blade has a light source that illuminates the inside of the mouth; the blade is used to pull the epiglottis down, exposing the opening of the trachea. Endotracheal tubes vary in length and diameter to accommodate most patient tracheal sizes. The endotracheal tube should have a slightly narrower diameter than the patient's trachea; however, should not be so small as to restrict breathing. Endotracheal widths are measured in millimeters and range in size from 2.0mm to 30mm. Endotracheal tubes, commonly used for dogs and cats, range in size from 3.0mm to 12mm.

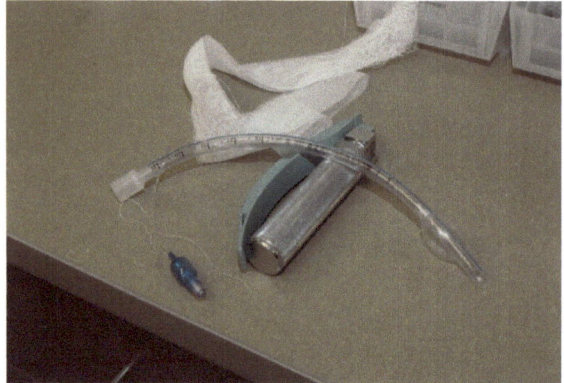

Figure 101: Laryngoscope and endotracheal tube

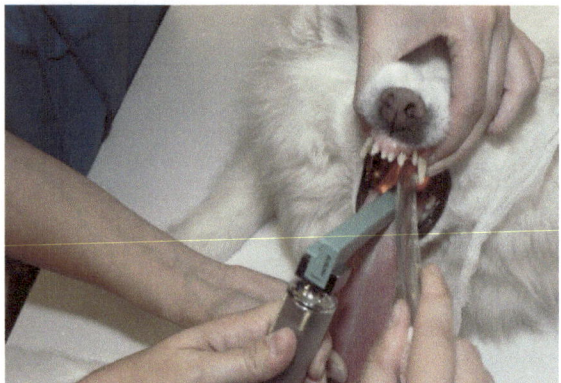

Figure 102: Intubation of a dog

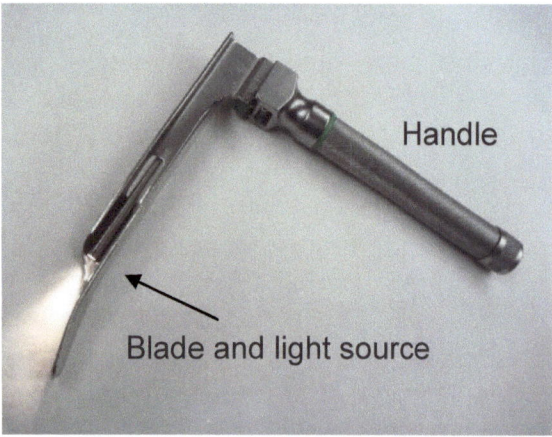

Figure 103: Laryngoscope

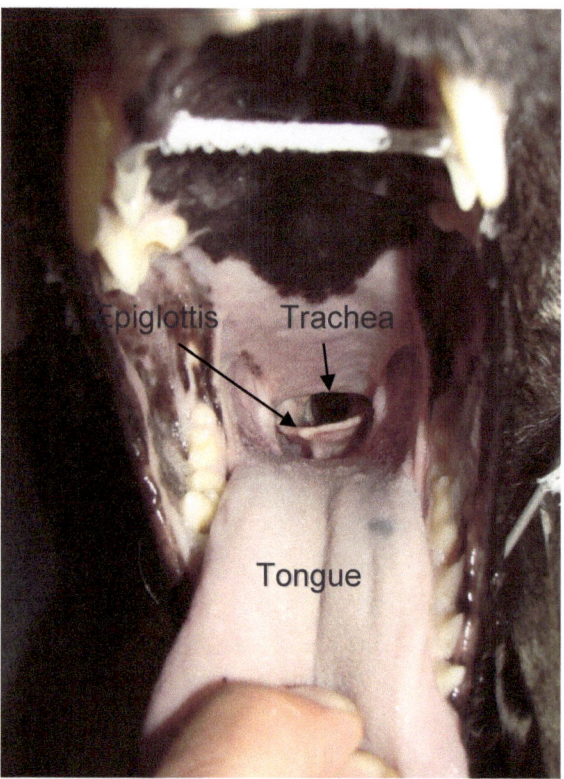

Figure 104: Oropharynx of the dog showing epiglottis and trachea

Chemical anesthetic drugs produce their effects on the body for varying lengths of time. In longer surgical procedures, anesthetic gases are sometimes used to maintain anesthesia. These gases are delivered to the patient through the anesthetic machine by the use of a precision anesthetic vaporizer. Gas anesthetics are liquid at room temperature, and require the use of a vaporizer to accurately deliver the gaseous form of these anesthetics to the patient. Anesthetic vaporizers require periodic refilling and are color coded to ensure that they are filled with the proper liquid anesthetic. Gas anesthetics can be administered to the patient via the endotracheal tube or with an anesthetic mask. The anesthetic mask allows more gas to escape, because of the inferior seal, and increases the exposure to veterinary staff.

Anesthetic	Color on vaporizer and anesthetic bottle
Halothane	Red
Isoflurane	Purple
Sevoflurane	Yellow
Desflurane	None-special filling cap

Table 21: Gas Anesthetic Color Codes

The Anesthetic Machine

The anesthetic machine delivers precise amounts of anesthetic gas and oxygen to the patient. One hundred percent medical grade oxygen is supplied to the anesthetic machine by use of a supply line (usually colored green) from an oxygen tank. Oxygen gas passes through a flow meter; oxygen flow can be adjusted based on the patient's needs.

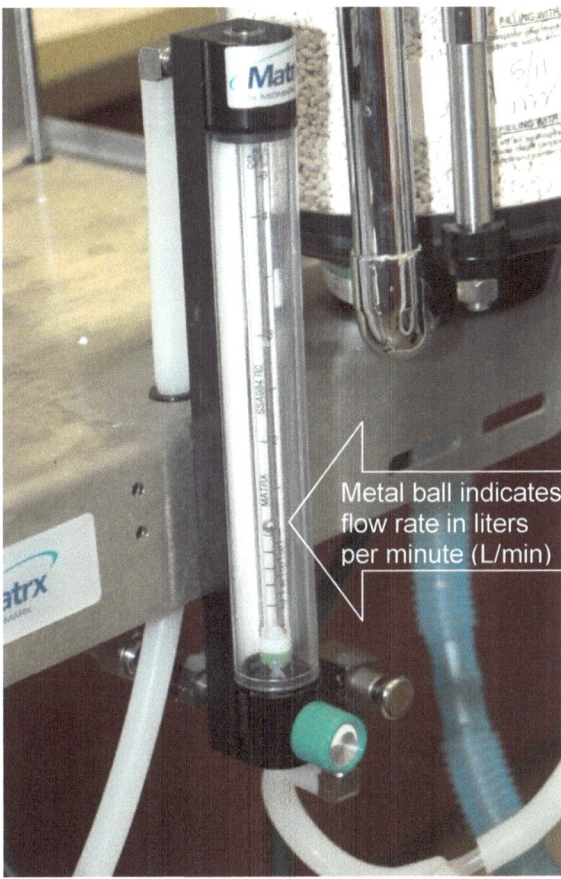

Metal ball indicates flow rate in liters per minute (L/min)

Figure 105: Oxygen flow meter

Oxygen flows to the vaporizer and anesthetic gas is mixed into the oxygen. The patient breathes in the oxygen/anesthetic mixture to establish or maintain anesthesia. Precision vaporizers have a dial that can be adjusted so precise amounts of anesthetic gas can be given to the patient. The amount is usually represented as a percentage of anesthetic agent. When the patient exhales, excess oxygen, anesthetic gas and carbon dioxide (CO_2) are removed by the use of a scavenging system.

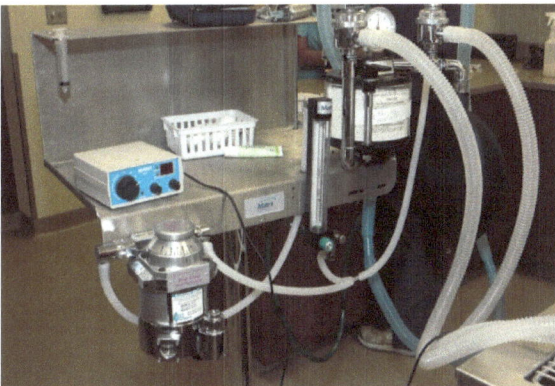

Figure 106: Small animal anesthetic machine

Scavenging systems can either be passive, where excess gasses leave by pressure, or active, where they are vacuumed away. Passive systems utilize a carbon filled canister that removes excess anesthetic gases from the other gases. This ensures that the veterinary staff is not exposed to scavenged anesthetic gases. Anesthetic machines have the ability to allow a patient to re-breathe exhaled anesthetic gases, except for CO_2, as it is a toxic gas. A re-breathing circuit passes exhaled anesthetic gases from the patient to a container of CO_2 absorbing granules. Once the CO_2 is removed, the patient may re-breath the gas mixture. Re-breathing systems conserve oxygen, anesthetic gas and heat from the patient. The white CO_2 absorbing granules turn purple when exhausted; this color change determines when to replace the granules.

Location	Gas	Example
Scavenging	Anesthetic	f-air canister
Re-breathing	CO_2	Baralyme Soda-sorb

Table 22: Examples of gas removing products

Two common anesthetic circuit systems are used in small animal veterinary practices; they include the non-re-breathing system and semi-closed re-breathing system. Patient size is the main determining factor when selecting one of these circuit systems, as air flow resistance is different with these two types of circuits. In general, the non-re-breathing system is designed for small patients weighing less than about 7kg and the re-breathing system is for those of greater weight. Both circuit systems have a reservoir bag that can be used to produce positive pressure ventilations to the patient, if necessary.

Monitor	Abbreviation	Function
Pulse Oximeter	SpO_2	Measures pulse rate and oxygen saturation
Capnograph (end tidal CO_2)	$ETCO_2$	Measures CO_2 concentration of expired air and respiration rate
Non-invasive blood pressure	NIBP	Measures blood pressure
Electro-cardiograph	ECG	Records electrical conduction of the heart

Table 23: Common Anesthetic Monitors

Anesthetic Monitoring

There are inherent risks with anesthesia. These risks are minimized by pre-anesthetic patient evaluation and organ function tests, as well as the use of monitoring equipment during anesthesia. Monitoring should also include experienced anesthetists who are able to identify early warning signs of anesthetic problems. A list of common anesthetic monitors can be found in table 23.

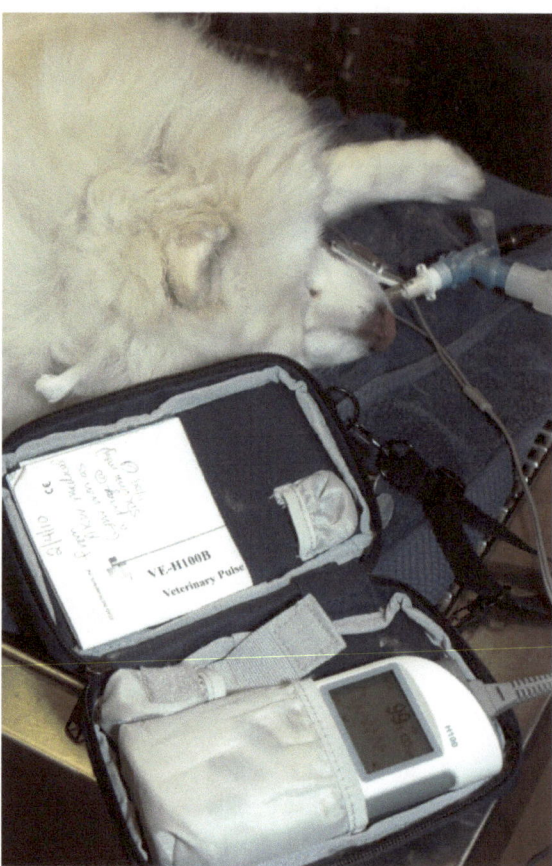

Figure 107: Pulse oximeter

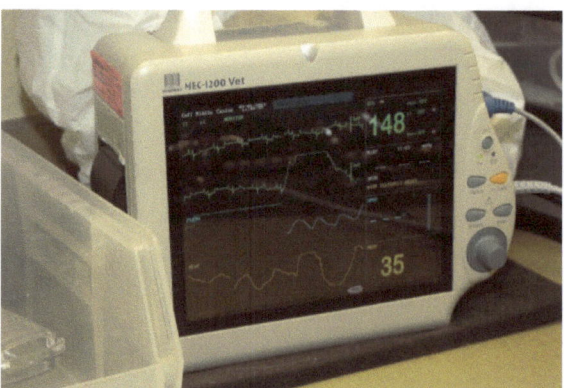

Figure 108: Multiparameter patient monitor

Anesthetic complications and emergencies happen infrequently. Patient monitoring is an important way to minimize anesthetic related emergencies.

Post Anesthetic Recovery

Patient monitoring should not end with the end of surgery; it should continue through the recovery stage. Patients will be uncoordinated, disorientated and compromised during this period. Patients will be hypersensitive to most stimuli, including light and noise. Care should be taken to minimize these stimuli in order to optimize a patient's smooth recovery. A dark, dimly lit recovery area is ideal. Most patients have lost heat during the anesthetic procedure, so it is important to provide supplemental heat. Periodical monitoring of vital signs such as respiration rate and heart rate will help to ensure patient wellness during recovery. Post surgical nausea is not uncommon and vomiting may occur. It is important to ensure that a patient has not aspirated or occluded its airway as a result of vomiting. Some patient's may have a nystagmus, or a bilateral horizontal twitching of the eyes; this should be considered normal if temporary, and is likely caused by the anesthetic drugs used. Some pet's may also cry and howl as they recover.

Post Anesthesia Complications

In addition to common side effects of anesthesia, some patient's may experience less common surgery related complications. Bleeding or oozing at the surgical site may be considered normal, but should be evaluated by the surgeon. Excessive hemorrhage at the surgical site is not normal. Wound dehiscence, or the failure of a wound to stay closed, may occur immediately or at some point in the surgical healing process. This complication is sometimes caused by obsessive licking of the surgical site. Analgesic medication may reduce this behavior, but sometimes an Elizabethan collar may be needed. Elizabethan collars, also known as e-collars, are plastic 'lamp-shades' that prevent the patient from reaching most surgical sites; thus, preventing the licking behavior. Anti-lick products such as Chew Guard can be applied to surgical sites. These products impart an unpleasant taste for the lick-motivated patient. Non-absorbable skin sutures may cause a local reaction; most are removed ten to fourteen days after surgery and require no intervention. Infection is a latent surgical complication affecting some pets. Infection may present in the form of local redness at the surgical site, abscessation, oozing and patient hyperthermia. Antibiotics may be prescribed, and the client may be asked to place a warm compress on the pet's surgical site daily until it is resolved.

Hematology and Urinalysis

Hematology is the study of blood, blood products and blood diseases. Hematological information, obtained from a patient, can be valuable in diagnosis of disease. The primary hematological evaluations performed in a veterinary practice include the complete blood count (CBC) and biochemical analysis (Chemistry). The CBC is used to identify the cellular composition of the blood, and the chemistry panel evaluates the non-cellular components including electrolyte values and organ functions. The CBC/chem can be performed in the veterinary practice with the use of in-house diagnostic analysis equipment. These compact machines can evaluate blood cell numbers, as well as chemical values. An in-house blood panel can be processed in less than one hour. There are several outside laboratories that provide diagnostic hematology services. Couriers pick up samples from the veterinary practices daily, and results are ready the following morning. Examples include Antech and Idexx laboratories.

Basic Laboratory Blood Tests
Several blood evaluations can be made in-house with relatively little equipment. These tests may provide quick and valuable information for the veterinarian. *Packed cell volume* or PCV test is used to determine the red blood cell component of blood. A micro-capillary tube is filled with whole blood and spun in a centrifuge. The centrifuge forces the heavier cells to the bottom of the tube, leaving the non-cellular portion on top. A

measuring device can be used to determine the proportion or percentage of red blood cells in the sample.

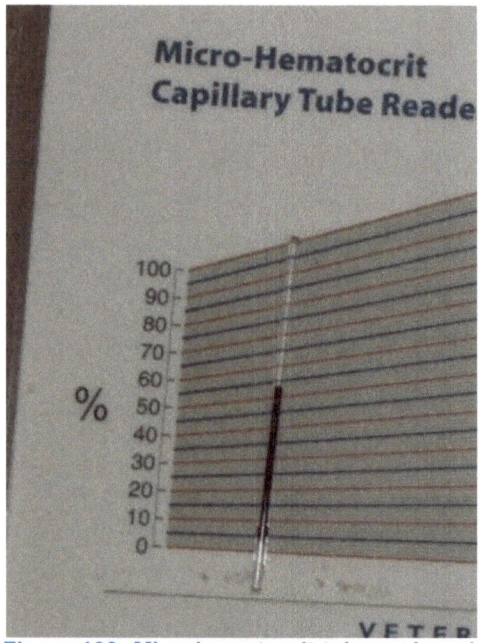

Figure 109: Microhematocrit tube and reader showing a PCV of 52%

The PCV is used to determine if a reduction of red blood cells or anemia is present. The value can also be determined with a ruler.

$$\frac{\text{Red blood cell length}}{\text{Total sample length}} \times 100 = \text{PCV percent}$$

The *total protein*, also known as the plasma protein (PP) of the non-cellular portion, can be determined by the use of a refractometer. A refractometer evaluates the solute concentration of liquids. Solutes distort or bend light in fluids; the more solutes present, the more the light is bent. The solute concentration of distilled water, therefore, should be zero. This is indicated by a blue field at the bottom of the scale (see figure 111). By placing a drop of plasma on the prism of the refractometer, the total protein can be determined.

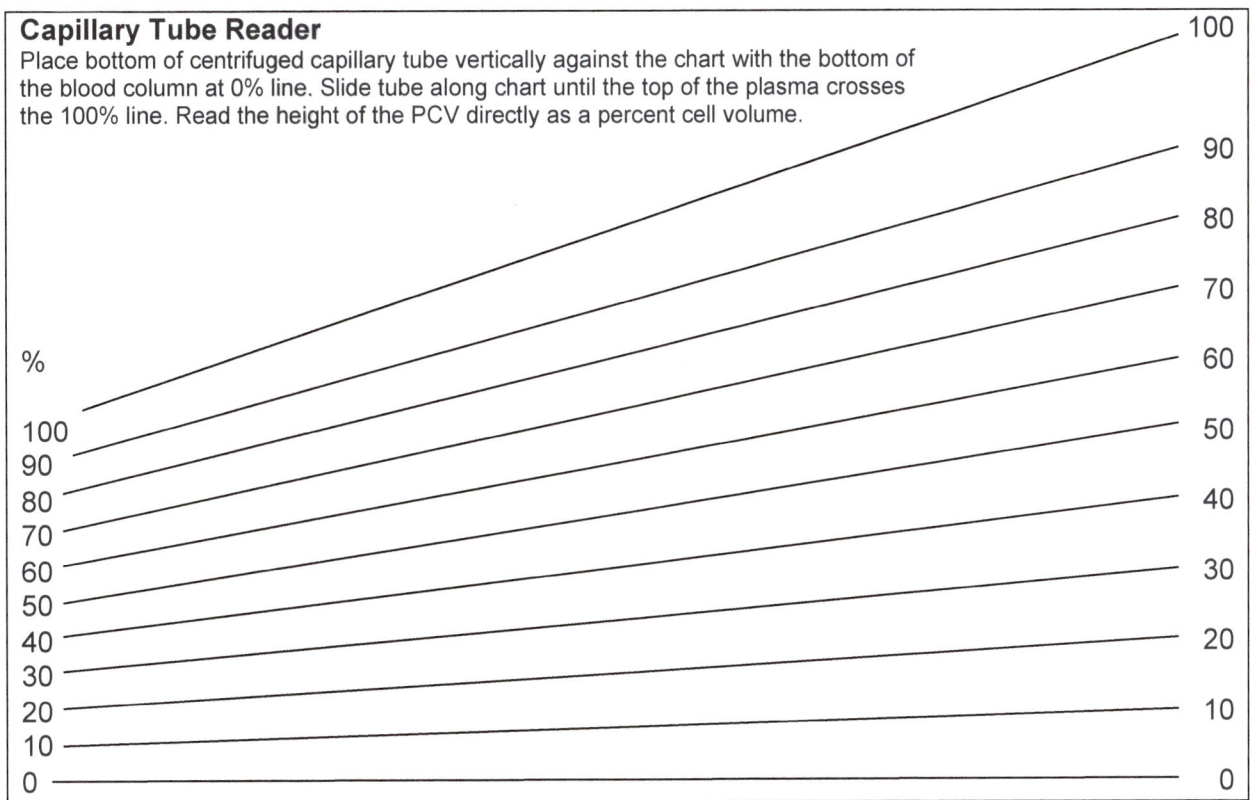

Capillary Tube Reader

Place bottom of centrifuged capillary tube vertically against the chart with the bottom of the blood column at 0% line. Slide tube along chart until the top of the plasma crosses the 100% line. Read the height of the PCV directly as a percent cell volume.

Figure 110: Capillary Tube Reader

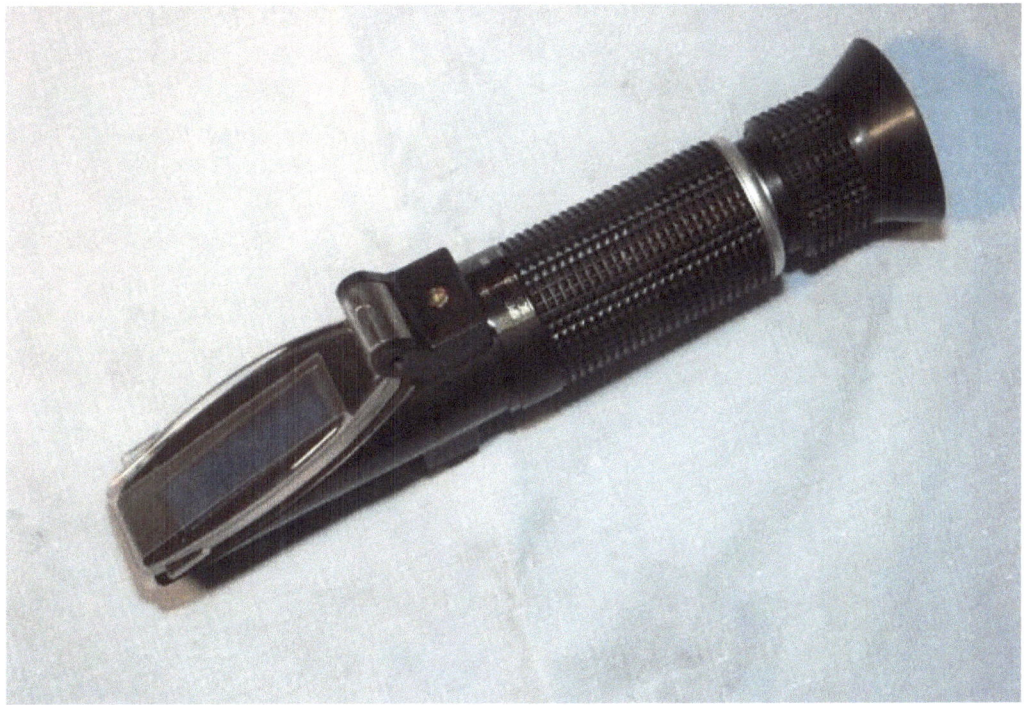

Figure 111: Refractometer

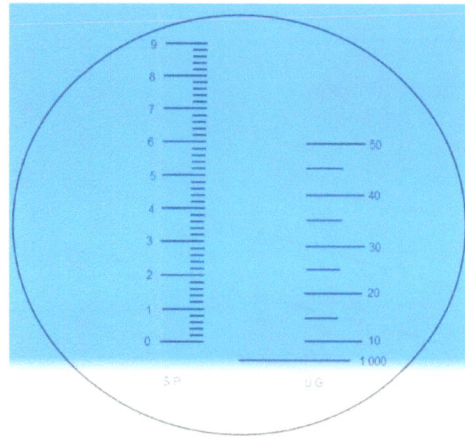

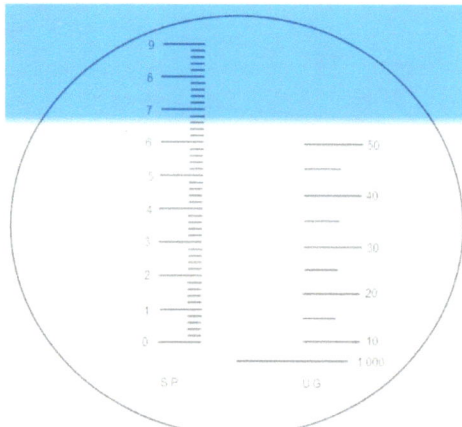

Figure 112: Refractometer eyepiece scale showing zero value of distilled water (top), and a serum protein level of 6.8

Blood urea nitrogen or BUN, is an indicator of kidney function. Nitrogen is abundant in nature in the body: therefore, it is constantly being eliminated. If the kidneys are functioning poorly, nitrogen containing compounds such as urea will accumulate in the blood. BUN is evaluated from blood with the use of a simple test strip. Blood is applied to the strip, and after sixty seconds its color change can correlate to predetermined values.

Blood Sample Handling
When blood is collected from a patient, it is put into blood tubes. These tubes are storage containers for the blood. Vacutainer blood tubes come in a variety of sizes and types. These tubes have a vacuum inside the tube equal to the amount of blood the tube holds; this makes filling the tube effortless as blood is actually sucked into the tube. The caps on the tubes are made of plastic or rubber and can be easily pierced with a needle. When the needle is removed, the tube remains sealed. Some tubes contain special liquids or powders that are designed to preserve the blood or prevent it from clotting. Some tubes have wax inside; this helps separate the cells from the non-cellular components when centrifuged. Blood samples collected for complete blood counts must not be clotted; whereas, chemistries can be run from clotted or unclotted samples. Blood can be stored in the refrigerator until they are processed or sent to an outside laboratory.

Blood Tube Types
The *green top tube* contains the anticoagulant, heparin. Heparin, a nature compound found in the body, prevents fibrinogen and platelets from binding and forming clots. Most green top tubes used in veterinary practices contain lithium heparin; however, sodium heparin can also be used. Heparinized tubes are commonly used for avian and reptile hematology.

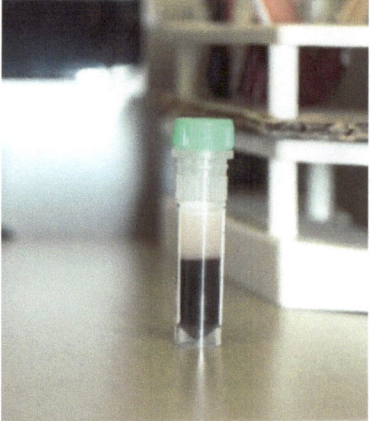

Figure 113: Heparinized blood tube (green top)

The *purple top tube* contains the anticoagulant ethyldiamine acetic acid (EDTA). This is the preferred tube for mammalian CBC's.

The *serum separator tube* (SST) is also called a tiger top tube. These tubes contain no anticoagulant and therefore clotting will occur. The tubes often contain a wax separator; this separates the heavier cells from the lighter serum. The SST is the preferred tube for mammalian chemistry evaluation.

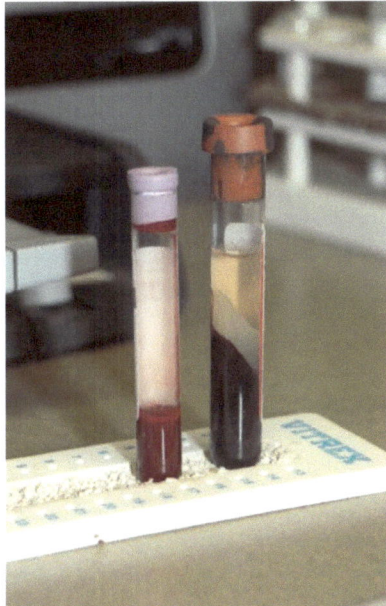

Figure 114: Purple top tube (left) and serum separator tube

Other tube types
The *royal blue top tube* is a sterile plastic tube used for mineral tests that are affected by rubber.

The *light blue top tube* is used for clotting time evaluation.

The *yellow top tube* contains ACD, an acid-citrate-dextrose preservative and nutrient to preserve cells.

Blood sample quality can be affected by collection technique. Poor phlebotomy technique can lead to sample clotting and hemolysis. Vigorous agitation of blood samples or excessive time to collect samples can lead to poor sample quality.

Blood products should be refrigerated until processed or sent to an outside laboratory. Cold packs and containers should be used when shipping biomedical samples such as blood products.

Tube color	Additive	Use
Green	Heparin	CBC
Purple	EDTA	CBC
Tiger top	None	Chemistry
Yellow	ACD	Transfusion
Royal blue	None	Minerals
Light blue	Citrate	Clotting time

Table 24: Common Blood Tube Colors and Uses

The Composition of Blood

Blood is composed of cells and a fluid matrix in which the cells are bathed. Blood cells include red blood cells (RBC's), white blood cells (WBC's), and platelets. RBC's, also known as erythrocytes, function to transport oxygen to the tissues of the body. They are round cells with a central pallor. RBC's constitute about ninety-five percent of the cellular components of blood.

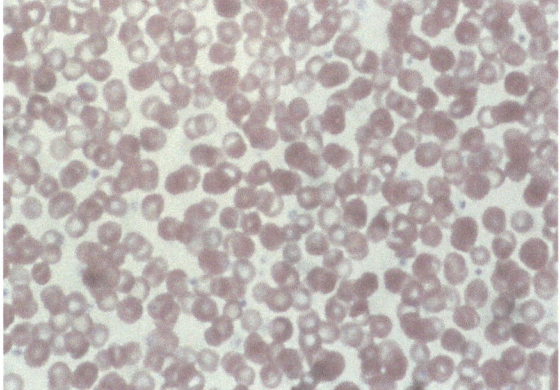

Figure 115: Normal blood, RBC's

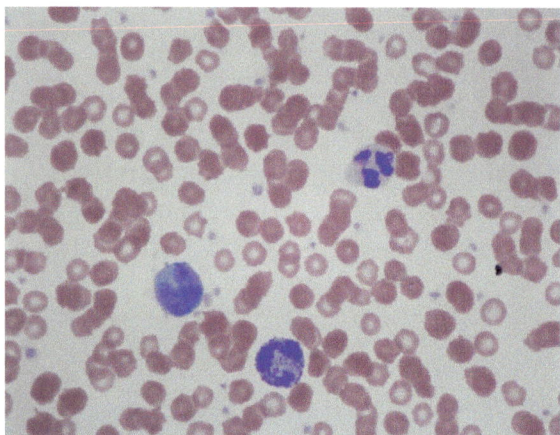

Figure 116: Normal blood, RBC's, Neutrophil, Monocyte and Basophil

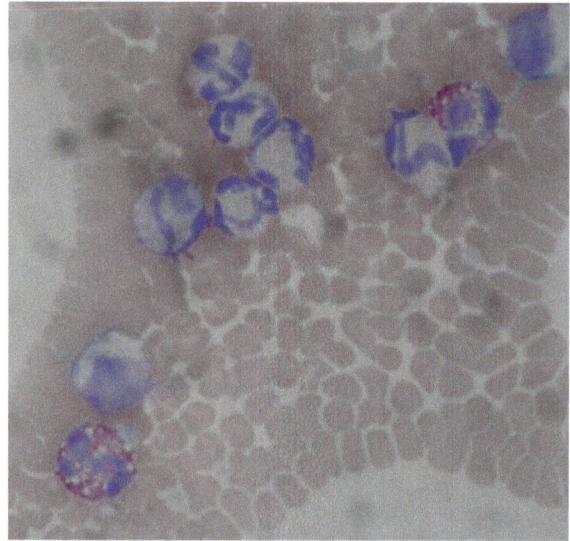

Figure 117: Several neutrophils, basophils and monocytes

WBC's, called leukocytes, function to fight infection and are responsible for the body's immune response. WBC's come in five distinct types. Each has a function in fighting infection. Neutrophils are the most prominent WBC in the body, making up sixty-five percent of all leukocytes. Neutrophils have a multilobed nucleus, and their increased numbers may indicate an infectious process. Lymphocytes are smaller, less prominent WBC's constituting forty percent of all leukocytes. These cells have a very small cytoplasm, making their nucleus look very large. Monocytes, also known as macrophages, are large phagocytic cells with polymorphic, multilobed nuclei. Basophils are involved with allergic and antigen response. These WBC's have a granular cytoplasm. Eosinophils are similar in appearance to basophils; however, their presence is suggestive of a parasitic infection.

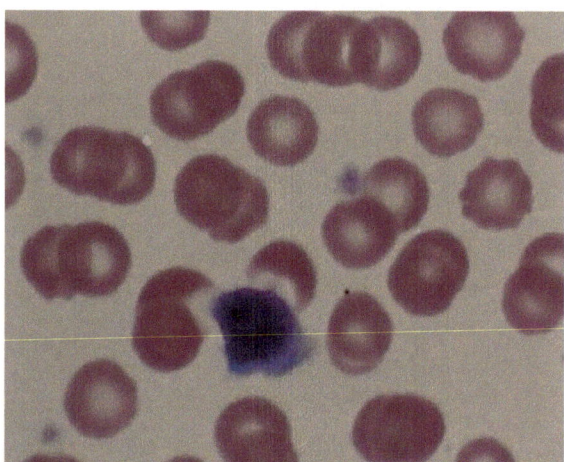

Figure 118: Normal blood, RBC's, platelets and a lymphocyte

Platelets are cells involved in the clotting process. They are very small in size, but are very important in the clotting cascade. When activated clotting factors, fibrinogen and platelets clump together and form a lattice. This lattice is the earliest stage of a clot.

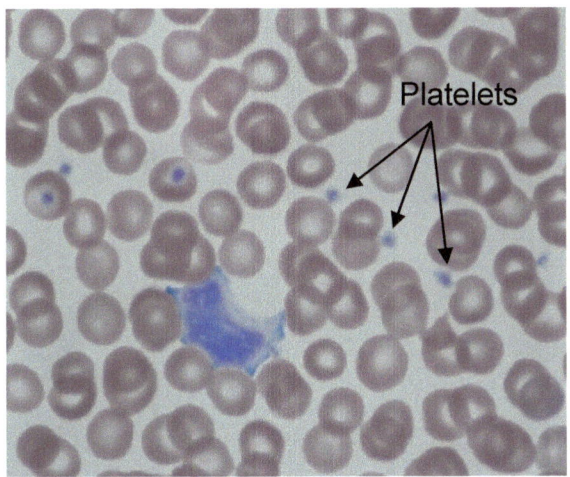

Figure 119: Normal blood, RBC's, monocyte and platelets

Cell type	Size (µm)	Numbers per (µl)
Erythrocyte	6-8	4-6 million
Neutrophil	10-12	
Lymphocyte	7-8	
Monocyte	14-17	
Basophil	12-15	
Eosinophil	10-12	
Platelet	2-3	150-400 thousand

Table 25: Blood cell types and sizes

The fluid portion of blood contains the following components:

- Water
- Nutrients
- Electrolytes
- Toxins and wastes
- Fibrinogen
- O_2
- CO_2
- Nitrogen

The CBC is determined from an unclotted blood sample; most are determined from a purple top tube. A heparinized green top tube can also be used. A hematocytometer is a special microscope slide used to quantify cell numbers and types in whole blood. The slide has gridlines on it, and allows a specific amount of blood in it. A small amount of blood is placed on the slide; cell types within the gridlines are counted, and values are determined based on percentages of cells observed. Automated cell counters can also be used to quantify a CBC. A blood smear can also be prepared and stained with dyes that penetrate the cells; cell types can then be evaluated.

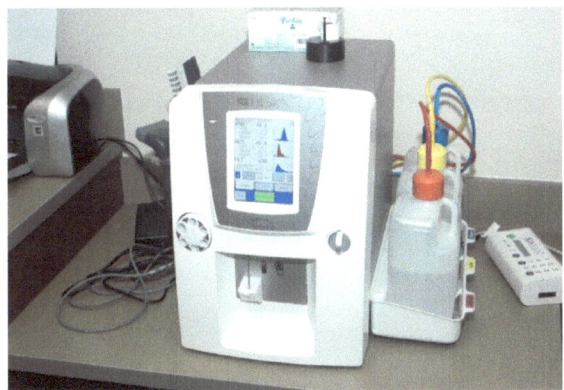

Figure 120: In house hematology machine

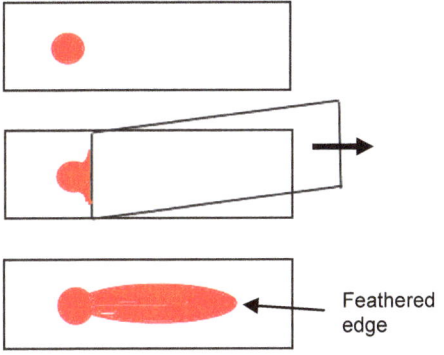

Feathered edge

Figure 121: Blood smear technique

A blood smear is made by placing a drop of whole (unclotted) blood on a slide. A second slide is placed atop of the first slide at a thirty-degree angle. The second slide is brought to the drop of blood, and then drawn away smearing the blood across the slide. The end of the smear, also known as the 'feathered edge', is where the blood cell composition is evaluated.

Chemistry analysis requires the use of the non-cellular component of blood. If the component is from non-clotted blood, it is called plasma. If the component is from clotted blood, it is called serum. The difference between plasma and serum is the presence or lack of fibrinogen, a clotting factor. Both serum and plasma are semi-clear liquids; any other color may be a result of abnormal conditions such as lipemia, jaundice, or hemolysis. These conditions may have an effect on chemistry values. In-house chemistry machines, as well as outside laboratories, can evaluate a multitude of tests on serum and plasma.

Drug levels, vaccine serology and antibody/antigen levels of many diseases can be determined from plasma and serum.

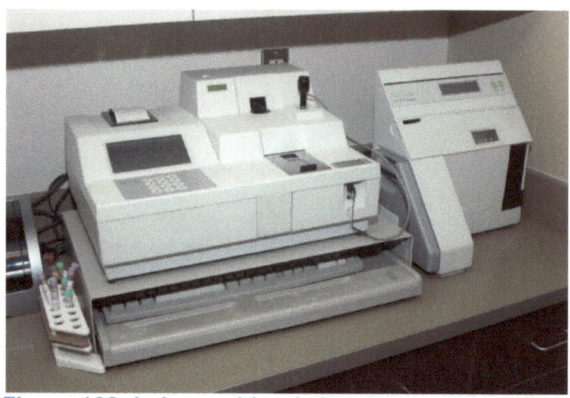
Figure 122: In house blood chemistry machine

Test	Evaluation
pH	Acid-base balance
Protein	Protein level
Glucose	Glucose level
ALT	Liver function
AST	Liver function
CPK	Muscle enzyme
Bilirubin	Liver function
Calcium	Mineral level
Sodium (Na)	Electrolyte balance
Potassium (K)	Electrolyte balance
BUN	Kidney function
Amylase/Lipase	Pancreatic function
T_4	Thyroid function

Table 26: Chemistry tests

A *urinalysis* is the evaluation of urine in the bladder. A urinalysis can determine the presence of bacteria, crystals, cells, and other elements that may indicate disease. Urine is generally collected in a sterile container or tube. A urine culture may be taken to identify the growth of bacterial elements. A culturette is used; it is generally a sterile cotton tipped applicator placed in a gel transport media. Urine cultures are generally not refrigerated after being collected. A urinalysis can be collected from the patient in several ways.

- Free catch
- Clean catch
- Urinary catheterization
- Cystocentesis

Free catch samples are obtained while the animal is urinating. This is the least invasive collection method for the pet; however, the sample may be contaminated by products in the urethra. Free catch samples can be difficult to collect if the patient is reluctant to urinate, or urinates quickly.

Clean catch samples are those collected off of the floor or other substrate. These floor samples are completely non-invasive for the pet, but can be highly contaminated by the environment. Floor samples are the least desirable urine collection method.

Urinary catheterization involves threading a plastic or rubber tube up the patient's urethra. This procedure can be very invasive however sample quality is generally good with little contamination from the urethra. Catheterization is generally successful even if the pet's bladder is nearly empty. Urinary catheterization is much easier to perform on a male patient than a female; the urethral opening in the female can be difficult to visualize and catheterize.

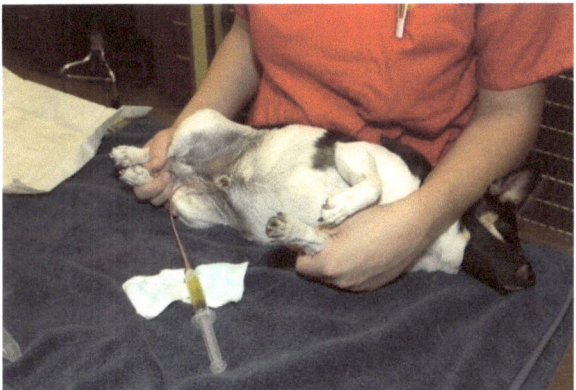

Figure 123: Urinary catheterization of a male dog

Cystocentesis involves the puncturing of the bladder with a syringe and needle through the abdomen. This method generally provides the best sample however is somewhat invasive to the patient. Patients are usually placed on their back for cystocentesis. The bladder is generally palpated prior to collecting the sample, although ultrasound guided cystocentesis can be used in patients with very small bladders. Cystocentesis is generally painless to the patient.

Evaluation of Urine
The first evaluation of a urine sample includes evaluation of specimen quality, clarity and odor. Many criteria and

descriptors of samples have been standardized for consistency purposes. Normal urine is generally yellow to orange in color, and clear in clarity. Odors can indicate infection, ingestion of certain foods, as well as gender specific fragrances. These odors, such as those common with tomcat urine, are generally used for scent marking, and are considered normal.

Color	Clarity	Odor
Yellow	Clear	Foul
Orange	Hazy	Pungent
Red	Cloudy/turbid	
	Hematuric	

Table 27: Common terms describing urine

Basic Laboratory Urine Tests
The *specific gravity* (SG) of urine can be determined with a refractometer. The function of the kidneys is to remove wastes, and concentrated urine being eliminated. Normal urine specific gravity is around 1.045; the specific gravity of distilled water is 1.000 on the refractometer scale. Diluted urine may have a specific gravity as low as 1.010. A low specific gravity may indicate renal failure.

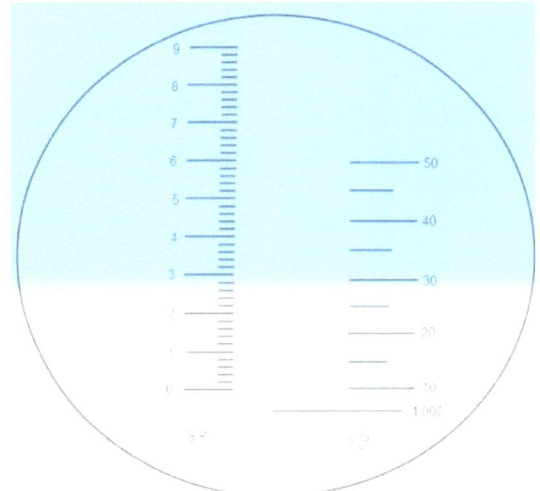

Figure 124: Refractometer eyepiece showing a urine specific gravity (UG) of 1.028

The *urine dip stick* or multistick, can be used to evaluate a multitude of tests including: protein, glucose, ketone, bilirubin, bacteria and blood levels. Urine is dripped on the multistick, and after 60 seconds, color changes on the strip can be compared to colors on the container. These colors reference numerical values that can then be interpreted.

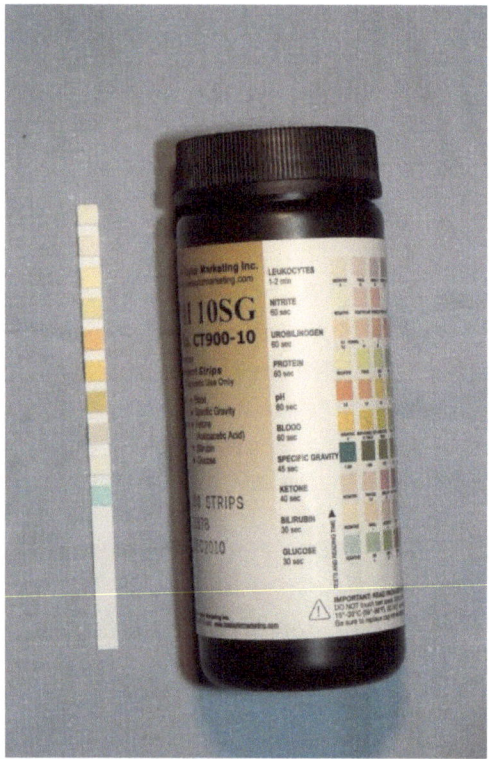

Figure 125: Urine multistix

Urine sediment can be evaluated. A small urine sample is spun in a centrifuge. The urine is spun for about 5 minutes, after which, the supernatant is poured off leaving the sediment in the bottom of the tube. A drop of sedi-stain is mixed with the sediment and poured onto a microscope slide. Sediment findings may include: epithelial cells, blood cells, bacteria, casts, crystals and debris.

Pharmacology

Pharmacology is the study of drugs, their history, physical and chemical properties, as well as their effects and actions. Pharmaceutical drugs can be considered any chemical agent that affects physiological processes. A target tissue is the site of a drugs action. Drugs are metabolized, degraded, transformed, and excreted by the body. The half life of a drug is the time required for a drug to decrease its serum concentration by 50%. A toxic or lethal dose of a drug can occur, and is considered a dose that exceeds the upper limit of a therapeutic dose.

Drug routes (refer to routes of administration, page 61)

Route	Also known as:
Enteral	Oral
Parenteral	SQ, IM, IV
Topical	Skin, eyes, ears

Table 28: Common Drug Routes

Drug Metabolism

Most drug metabolism occurs in the liver. The process of metabolism causes drugs to be bio-transformed into an inactive form of the drug over time. Some drugs; however, can be administered in an inactive form and be bio-transformed into the desired active form of the drug. Drug metabolism can also occur in the small intestine, kidneys, the brain and lungs. Dysfunction of any of these organs can affect the ability for drugs to be metabolized. In some cases, blood tests are required to evaluate organ function prior to or during the use of some medications.

Excretion
Drugs are usually excreted by the kidneys, while other drugs can be excreted through the lungs and digestive system.
Drug excretion is affected by kidney dysfunction.

Drugs can be grouped into classes based on their primary function. For example, Enrofloxacin and penicillin are types of antibiotics. Drugs within these groups are generally chosen because of veterinarian preference, because of its mode of administration, its efficacy, or because of side effects or interactions with other drugs. A list of commonly used veterinary drugs, classes and indications for use can be found in table 29.

Nutraceuticals

Nutritional substances that have effectiveness in the body similar to pharmaceuticals can be termed nutraceuticals. These non-drug substances are produced from foods, but are marketed in a medicinal form. Nutraceuticals are not subject to the same FDA scrutiny and government regulations that pharmaceuticals must adhere. One concern with nutraceuticals is the potential of varied concentrations of the product because of the lack of regulations.
Glucosamine, a joint supplement and omega 3, a fatty acid, are commonly used nutraceuticals in some veterinary practices.

Class	Use	Example
Analgesics	Pain relief	Buprenorphine Butorphanol Tramadol
Antibiotics	Treat infection	Enrofloxacin Amoxicillin Trimethoprim-sulfa Clavamox
Diuretics	Water loss	Furosemide
Steroids	Anti-inflammatory	Prednisone Dexamethasone
NSAIDs	Non Steroidal anti-inflammatory	Meloxicam Ketoprofen Phenylbutazone
Cardio-vascular	Vasoconstriction Vasodilatation Contractility Arrhythmias	Atropine Ephedrine Digitalis Lidocaine
Antiparasitics	Deworming	Piperazine Fenbendazole Pyrantel Ivermectin Praziquantel Pyrethrin
Antifungals	Treat fungal infections	Itraconazole
Hormones	Treat hormone deficiencies	Levothyroxine Oxytocin Insulin
Antiemetics	Inhibit vomiting	Metoclopramide
Emetics	Induce vomiting	Apomorphine

Table 29: Commonly used drugs, classes and uses

Pharmaceutical medications may require a prescription or be available over the counter without a prescription. Prescription medications are drugs that require a prescription because they are considered harmful if not used under the supervision of a doctor. Some prescription drugs have additional controls placed on them. These drugs are called controlled or scheduled drugs. Controlled drugs are regulated based on their potential for abuse, addiction, or risk. In a veterinary practice, these drugs are kept in a locked cabinet, and a controlled drug record must be maintained. Controlled drugs are placed into schedules; those with the highest potential for abuse are placed in schedule I, and those with the lowest potential, in schedule V. Scheduled drugs may also be identified with a C-I, C-II, C-III, C-IV, or C-V. Some commonly used scheduled drugs in veterinary medicine include Ketamine, a dissociative anesthetic, Diazepam and Midazolam, both anxiolytic tranquilizers, Buprenorphine, an analgesic, Butorphanol, a barbiturate, and Phenobarbital, an antiepileptic. Pentobarbital, a schedule II controlled drug, is a barbiturate used for animal euthanasia.

Schedule	Risk of abuse	Examples
I	High	LSD, Heroin, Marijuana
II		Oxymorphone, Pentobarbital, Cocaine, Morphine, Amphetamine, Oxycodone
III		Vicodin, Ketamine, Buprenorphine
IV	Low	Diazepam, Midazolam, Phenobarbital, Butorphanol
V		Lomotil

Table 30: Scheduled Drugs

Controlled Drug Log

By law, controlled drug use and dispensing must be recorded in a controlled drug log. The log records the quantity of drugs being dispensed as well as the remaining balance. The Drug Enforcement Agency (DEA) enforces laws relating to controlled drug dispensing and record keeping.

Anesthesia log

Anesthesia logs are used to record anesthetic procedures, drugs used, as well as the duration of anesthetic time. Many of the drugs used for anesthetic induction and maintenance are scheduled drugs; an anesthetic log adds a source of redundancy to the recording requirements of controlled substances.

Computer software and databases have streamlined the way pharmaceuticals are recorded and inventoried. Veterinary practice management programs enable veterinary facilities to record and track medication use and inventory. This is an effective means to monitor inventory and re-ordering needs. By tracking medication supply and use, veterinary practices can have an appropriate supply of medication on hand without an excessive overstock that may expire if not utilized.

Veterinary facilities generally buy medications from drug companies and distributers in bulk. Most prescriptions can be filled with a fraction of a 'stock' bottle of medication. When a prescription is filled and dispensed from a veterinary practice, the medications are placed in a pharmacy container. These containers, similar to prescription drugs obtained from a drug store, must contain appropriate information about the prescription on the bottle. Label requirements for a prescription bottle include:

- Name, address, and telephone number of clinic
- Name of client
- Animal identification
- Species of animal
- Date prescription is dispensed
- Prescribing veterinarian
- Name of medication
- Quantity of medication dispensed
- Directions (script)
- Number of refills

Auxiliary labels may include user information such as:

- Shake well
- Keep refrigerated
- Protect from light

Organization of the Veterinary Pharmacy

Most veterinary practices stock prescription medications for in-hospital use or for dispensing to patients; some practices may have clients use human pharmacies to fill some medications. Many medications used in veterinary medicine are similar or identical to those stocked in human pharmacies.

Medications in a veterinary pharmacy can be organized in a multitude of ways.

Drug Form

This organizational system places all forms of drugs together. For example, all tablets and capsules are grouped together, followed by liquids and injectables.

Drug class

By grouping all classes of drugs together, such as antibiotics, the veterinarian can see all available medications in that class, and select the most desirable drug for the situation.

Alphabetical

Alphabetizing drugs by form or class is common. Additionally, some practices may alphabetize their entire inventory without regard to form or class.

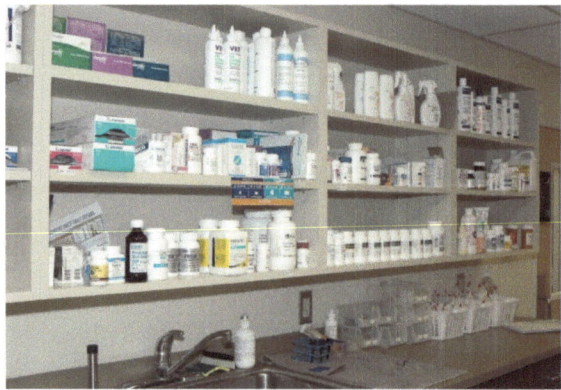

Figure 126: Veterinary hospital pharmacy

Generic and Brand Name Drugs

All drugs have several names. This includes the chemical name, common or generic name, and the brand name. The chemical name describes the drug composition. The common or generic name is often a function of its chemical name in whole or parts. The brand name is given by the manufacturer, and may include the common name, or reference what the drug does. Brand names may help make the drug more attractive and marketable.

Molecular structure	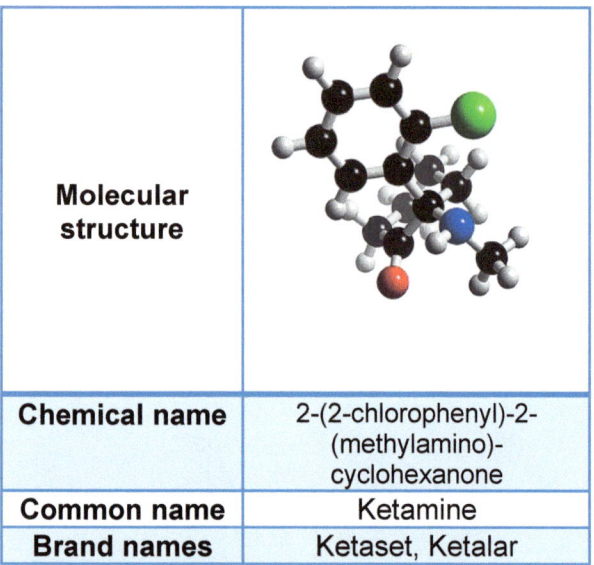
Chemical name	2-(2-chlorophenyl)-2-(methylamino)-cyclohexanone
Common name	Ketamine
Brand names	Ketaset, Ketalar

Table 31: Drug name and composition of Ketamine

Disposal of Medications

Drug disposal may be regulated by individual states, and is intended to reduce the impact drugs have on the environment. By imposing proper methods of disposal, expired and disposed medications will not contaminate soil or water supplies. Medications, usually in the form of expired drugs, should be disposed of in a biological waste container. This method of disposal is used to reduce environmental contamination in landfills and water supplies. Medication waste disposal companies charge the client, based on the weight of the medication being disposed. Controlled drugs disposal is regulated by the DEA, and disposal records must be kept for at least two years.

MSDS

Every drug, pharmaceutical, and chemical used in a veterinary practice must have a material safety data sheet, or MSDS. Material safety data sheets have information about drugs, including the manufacturer, chemical name, exposure levels and limits, physical properties, health hazards and reactivity. This information can assist the veterinary team in the proper handling, safe use, and properties of all drugs and chemicals used in the clinic. Material safety data sheets must be placed in a readily accessible area of the veterinary clinic. MSDS information can also be found online at http://www.msds.com/ .

PDR

The Physicians' Desk Reference is a publication that lists drugs by the manufacturer, generic and brand names. The book also includes illustrations of drugs for identification purposes. The PDR is designed for human drugs, and may not contain veterinary drugs.

USP

United States Pharmacopeia is a non-government public standards-setting authority for prescription and over the counter medicines. USP also sets standards for food ingredients and supplements.

Dentistry

Dental care is an important component of a pets healthcare. Routine dental evaluation and prophylaxis (cleaning) should be a consideration for all pets. Just as with people, poor dental hygiene in pets can lead to gingivitis and periodontal disease.

The tooth is comprised of the root and enamel covered crown. Depending on the type, the tooth may be used for crushing, tearing, or piercing food items. Teeth may also be used for grooming and defense. Tooth shapes vary based on their primary function, and may be flat, rounded or pointed. The crown of the tooth is generally smaller than the associated root, and therefore most of the tooth resides below the gingiva or gum line. Ligaments hold the tooth root into the jaw bone. The inside of the tooth contains a nerve and blood supply located in the pulp cavity. Mammals have two sets of teeth; deciduous or baby teeth, followed by permanent or adult teeth. As the adult teeth erupt from the jaw, they erode the deciduous teeth away, forcing them out. In some cases deciduous teeth do not come out and may need to be removed.

Teeth cleaning can be performed by a veterinary assistant, but dental extractions can only be performed by a DVM or RVT.

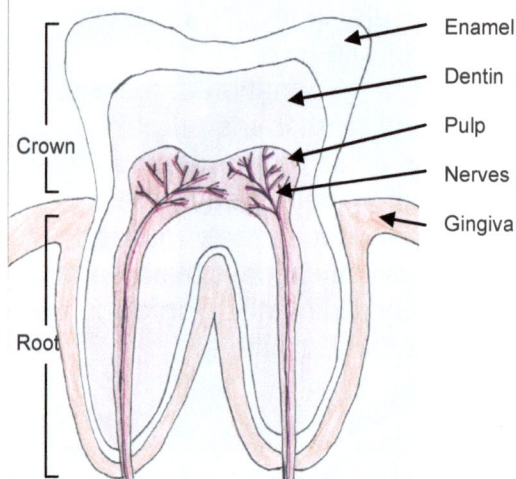

Figure 127: Anatomy of the tooth

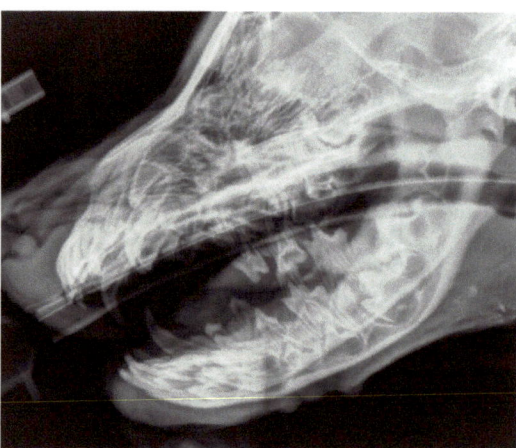

Table 32: Skull radiograph showing deciduous and adult dentition

Dogs and cats have four types of adult teeth; they include the incisors, canines, premolars and molars.

- *Incisors*-the small teeth in the front of the mouth
- *Canines*-large pointed teeth behind the incisors
- *Premolars*-large multi-rooted teeth behind the canines, and along the side of the mouth
- *Molars*-small teeth behind the premolars

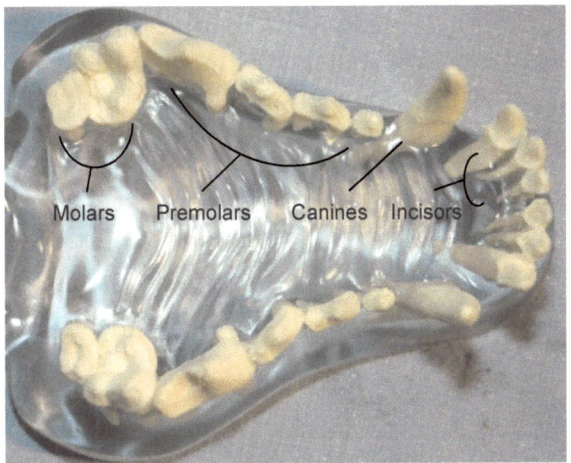
Figure 128: Upper dental arcade of the dog

Dental formulas are often used to describe the numbers and types of teeth for a given breed or species. The formula reflects the teeth on one side of the upper or maxillary arcade, and one side of the lower or mandibular arcade. Because the teeth are bilaterally symmetrical (same numbers of teeth on each side); the total number of teeth would be twice that of the dental formula. The general formula would appear as follows:

$$\frac{\text{Upper}}{\text{Lower}} \Longrightarrow \frac{I\ C\ P\ M}{I\ C\ P\ M} \times 2 = \text{Total teeth}$$

(I=incisor, C=canine, P=premolar, M=molar)

Breed	Adult Teeth	Formula
Dog	42	3 1 4 2 3 1 4 3
Cat	30	3 1 3 1 3 1 2 1

Figure 129: Dental formulas for dogs and cats

Dental Pathology
The accumulation of tartar can have profound effects on dental health. Dental tartar, or calculus, accumulates at the base of the tooth where the tooth meets the gingiva. This gingival sulcus can become inflamed as a result of the irritation from the tartar leading to gingivitis. Gingivitis is the earliest stage of dental disease and is characterized by gingival redness, swelling and bleeding. Periodontitis occurs as gingival recession occurs exposing the unprotected root of the tooth. As this continues, periodontal ligaments become compromised, infection develops, and teeth are lost. Cavities and tooth fractures can also lead to infections and tooth loss.

Dental Prophylaxis
Veterinary dental prophylaxis utilizes much of the same equipment as human dentistry. One significant difference is the use of general anesthesia to facilitate the cleaning. The use of anesthesia enables the dentistry to be performed safely and efficiently. Types of dental cleaning equipment include the hand scaler, ultrasonic and roto-scalers. Dental drills are generally air driven.

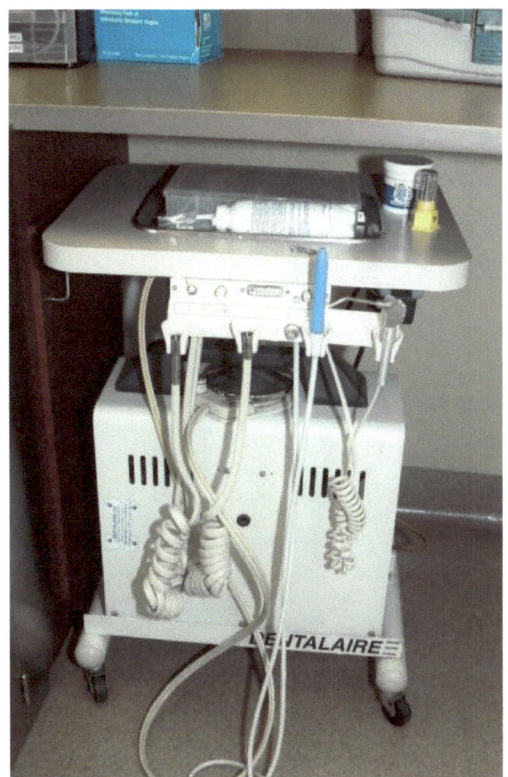
Figure 130: Air-driven dental machine

Hand scalers are often used to remove large pieces of tartar from the surface of the teeth. The hand piece tips are variable in style, but enable the veterinary dentist to chip away large pieces of tartar (calculus) or debris.

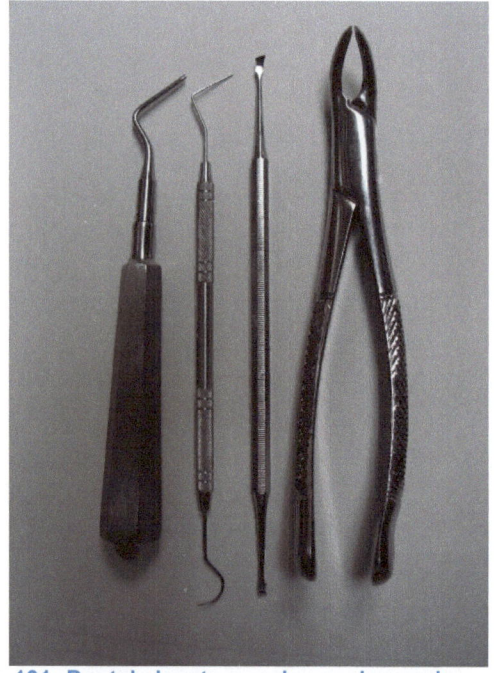

Figure 131: Dental elevator, probe, scaler, and extractor (left to right).

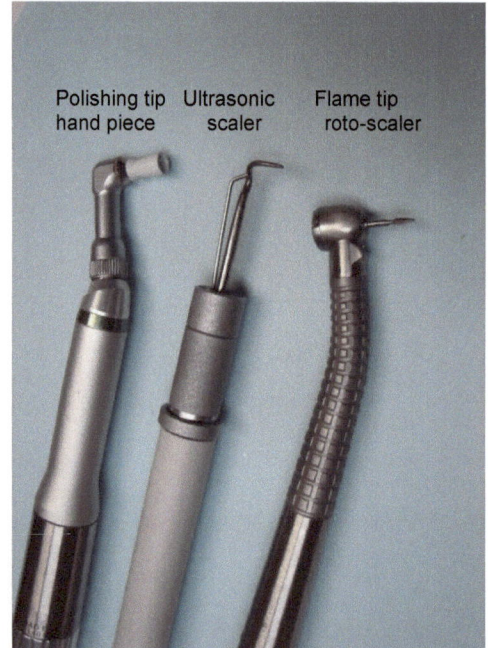

Polishing tip hand piece   Ultrasonic scaler   Flame tip roto-scaler

Figure 132: Various air-driven dental drills

Ultrasonic scalers utilize water and high frequency vibrations to dislodge tartar from the surface of the teeth. The water is used to counteract the heat generated from the scaler. The tip of the ultrasonic scaler can reach below the gum line and between teeth for superior cleaning. *The roto-scaler* has a flame tip that removes tartar by the concussion of its blunted bit on the teeth. Forced water is used to keep the teeth cool while the scaler is removing tartar. It is also essential that the roto-scaler be kept moving to ensure that the teeth are not damaged from heat or contact by the bit. Roto-scalers are effective in removing significant accumulations of tartar. Cup *polishing tips* are used to buff the teeth after the removal of any tartar. These low speed tips are used to apply a protective fluoride polish to the teeth.

Extractions may be indicated for teeth that are loose or have been compromised by periodontal disease. Hand held dental elevators and pliers are used for breaking down ligaments and attachments of the tooth being removed. Care is taken to remove the whole tooth including the roots. Because of the risk and skill required, dental extractions can only be performed by the veterinarian or veterinary technician.

Home dental care can include the use of dental tooth pastes, brushes and chew bones that are designed to reduce the buildup of tartar. Several dog and cat foods are available that are designed to aid in the management of dental tartar.

A root canal may be performed if a tooth root has been compromised but the tooth is still intact. The technique involves the removal of the tooth root with special files, cleaning and drying the exposed canal, and filling it with a durable composite material. Root canals may be done for esthetic reasons and can be more expensive than the extraction of the tooth.

Dental radiography is used to see the quality of tooth attachment to the jaw. Fractures and lytic areas can be seen in a dental radiograph.

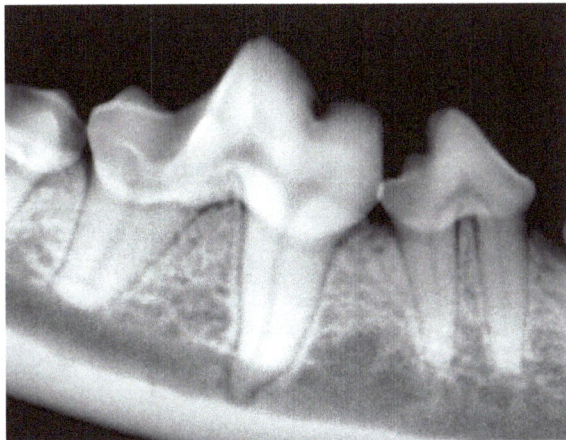

Figure 133: Dental radiograph showing premolars. Thanks to Boulders Natural Animal Hospital.

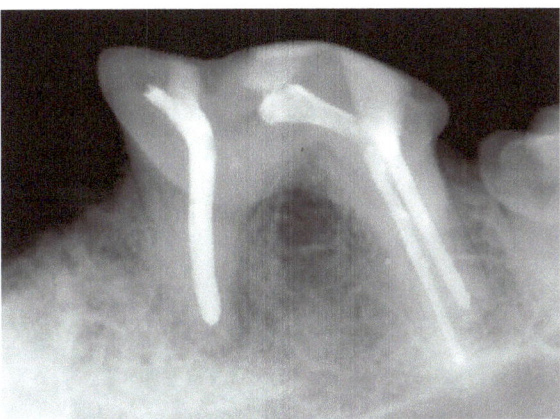

Figure 134: Dental radiograph showing root canal of a premolar. Thanks to Apex Veterinary Hospital.

Nutrition

Nutrition is an important component of pet health. Owners have a tremendous variety of pet food manufacturers and products available for their pets. The pet food industry spends time and money in research and product analysis to ensure it provides the proper nutrition for one's pet. Common companion animal pet food products include: canned, dry and semi-moist foods. Additionally, special diets are available to meet specific dietary needs or medical necessity. Some dog and cat foods are also designed for specific stages of a pet's life.

Pet food generally consists of meat, meat byproducts, cereals and grains. Pet foods may also include ingredients such as preservatives, artificial colors and stabilizers. Some additives or ingredients afford no nutritional value, and therefore cannot be considered a nutrient. A nutrient is a chemical used by the body to live and grow. The six basic nutrients include: proteins, fats, carbohydrates, vitamins, minerals and water.

Energy producing nutrients
- Proteins or amino acids found in meat, chicken and fish
- Fats or fatty acids from plants and animals
- Carbohydrates or sugars, starches, and fiber found in plants (High caloric)

Non-energy producing nutrients
- Vitamins are organic compounds essential to the body
- Minerals are generally needed in trace amounts and some are essential for metabolism
- Water is an essential nutrient and is necessary for all chemical reactions

Nutrient		Examples
Protein	Energy producing	Meat, poultry, fish, byproducts
Fat		Animal, and vegetable fats and oils
Carbohydrate		Plant sugars, starches, and fiber
Vitamin	Non-energy producing	Vitamins A, B, C, D, E, K
Mineral		Calcium, Sodium, Potassium
Water		

Table 33: The 6 basic nutrients

Anatomy of Dog and Cat Foods

Dog and cat food labels must contain a list of ingredients. Ingredients are listed in descending order based on their weight; therefore, those ingredients at the top of the list constitute the greatest weight. The guaranteed analysis provides information relating to the composition of the food. Crude protein, fat, fiber, and moisture are required to be listed.

Dry dog and cat foods contain as little as ten percent water, while canned foods contain upwards of seventy-five percent water. It is difficult to compare a wet food to a dry food, but it is suggested that wet foods contain more protein, moisture and vitamins. Even the most finicky eater will generally eat wet food. Canned foods contain fewer preservatives, have a shorter shelf life once opened, and tend to be more expensive. Dry kibble is generally more economical, and exercises the pets jaw muscles; it may help prevent the accumulation of dental tartar. Nutritionally, generic pet foods are similar to brand name pet foods. Differences in primary ingredients and quality may affect the amounts needed to be consumed for the same caloric value. It is always best to compare pet food labels and determine which is more nutritionally beneficial. In general, Brand name pet food will be more expensive than a generic brand.

Feeding Methods and Considerations

Many feeding strategies can be used for companion animals. These strategies are used to optimize feeding time, limit overeating and reduce waste.

Portion control is usually based on the manufacturers' recommendations; this is usually determined by the pet's weight. Adjustments to the portion can be made if food is left over. Portions can also be split into morning and evening feedings for example.

Free choice places the pet in charge of the amount and time in which food is available. This strategy, if not properly monitored, may lead to pet obesity, and just as with portion control, uneaten food may attract pests and other unwanted animals to the feeding area.

Time control gives the pet a finite amount of time to eat. This ensures that the pet eats in a timely manner, and prevents leftover food from being left out for others. Time control is beneficial in multi-pet households where one pet may be eating additional food due to dominance.

Feeding Puppies and Kittens

Most animals do a great job caring for their offspring and supplying them with the ideal form of nutrition during nursing. If assisted feeding is necessary,

however, there are products that can be used to 'replace' mother's milk. There are several manufacturers of milk replacers for dogs and cats. Made of goat's milk, milk replacers supply the nutritional needs of these neonatal pets. Puppies and kittens grow rapidly, and therefore require multiple feedings daily. Giving approximately two to four grams of milk replacer for every kilogram of body weight each day is common. Many neonates will nurse well with the use of a bottle and nipple; however, some may need the assistance of a gavage tube. Gavage tubes are threaded directly to the stomach ensuring that aspiration of the milk does not occur. Food and milk aspiration is a serious and potentially life threatening problem for assisted fed neonates. Weaning occurs between 3 to 5 weeks of age; at that time a transition to a hard food diet can occur.

Feeding Young and Active Pets

Once transitioned to a hard diet, puppies and kittens should be given a product rich in protein and calories for their active and growing bodies. These products, though marketed for young pets, can also be used for active adult pets. These foods often contain high levels of fat so careful evaluation of the pet's weight should be monitored. Additionally, once a pet has been spayed or neutered, their daily dietary requirement decreases by ten percent, therefore, feeding amounts recommended on the product being used should be adjusted.

Feeding Geriatric Pets

As a pet reaches its senior years of life, dietary changes will occur. These pets become less active and their ability to process and digest foods changes. Pet food manufacturers have recognized the dietary needs of these animals and have created products designed for geriatric or senior pets. These products contain protein of high biologic value to reduce metabolites. Dietary fats are digestible to reduce obesity. Elements such as phosphorus are limited to reduce the effects on the kidneys.

Prescription Diets

Some pets may require a special diet specific for the condition, disease or malady the pet is experiencing. Several pet food products are available that are designed to treat problems such as obesity, skin conditions, heart disease, and bladder infections. These products can be relatively expensive, but tend to be very effective.

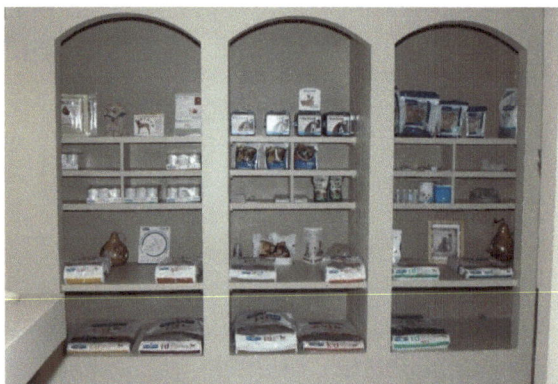

Figure 135: Display of veterinary diets

Raw Food Diets

The concept of feeding raw food to a pet has been extensively debated. Proponents of raw food diets contend that animals are meant to eat raw food, and look to their wild counterparts as an example. Pet food companies contend that processed dog and cat foods are nutritionally superior to raw diets and are more balanced. A significant concern with raw food diets is the possible exposure to the pet owner of salmonella that may be present in raw or undercooked meat.

Body Condition Scoring

Attempts to standardize the way veterinarians interpret body condition and weight has led to a body condition scoring system. This system ranks pets numerically from one to nine, based on their body condition. The presence or absence of body contours, ribs and spine, are all factors in determining a pet's body condition score. A pet of ideal condition would earn a body condition score of five; whereas, an obese pet would get a nine.

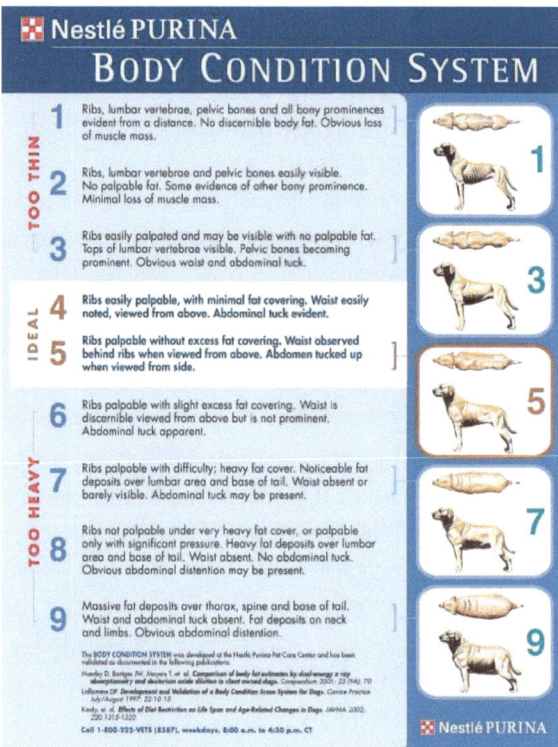

Figure 136: Nestle Purina body scoring system

Euthanasia

The term euthanasia originates from the Greek words eu, meaning good, and thantos, meaning death. Euthanasia refers to the humane termination of life. Pet euthanasia is a legal medical procedure in veterinary medicine. Animal overpopulation is an enormous problem. Over four million pets are euthanized in shelters every year. Other reasons for euthanasia include: biting and other behavioral problems such as house soiling and aggression. Unwanted and geriatric pets are sometimes euthanized for quality of life reasons. Divorce, moving, and finances are all reasons pets are euthanized.

Euthanasia is a Greek word meaning 'good death'.

Laws Regarding Euthanasia

By law, animal euthanasia must be performed humanely, with as little pain and distress to the animal as possible. The AVMA and IACUC, the Institutional Animal Care and Use Committee, outline humane animal practices including methods of euthanasia. IACUC is especially prominent in research.

By law, any pet being euthanized must not have bitten a person within ten days prior to the euthanasia. This is to ensure that the pet does not have rabies, and therefore protects the bite victim. The pet owner must sign a form to this effect.

The Process of Euthanasia

Euthanasia drugs for lethal injection in humans include the use of sodium thiopental, curare and potassium chloride (KCL). This combination of drugs depresses the central nervous system, paralyzes the muscles and stops the heart respectively. In veterinary medicine, sodium pentobarbital, a potent barbiturate, is used. Brand names include Euthasol, and Beuthanasia-D. These products are usually colored pink or blue to ensure that they are not confused with another drug. An overdose of sodium pentobarbital is given intravenously and causes rapid cardiac and respiratory arrest. Some veterinarians will give a sedative prior to euthanasia to ensure the pet is calm, relaxed and tolerant of the IV injection. In some cases, an IV catheter may be placed to facilitate ease of drug administration. It is not uncommon for a pet to have a respiratory sigh or muscle movement shortly after euthanasia; this is a reflexive process. The veterinarian will auscult or listen to the pet's heart after euthanasia to ensure that the pet is deceased. It is not uncommon for a pet to urinate or defecate as a result of sphincter muscle relaxation.

Other Modes of Euthanasia

Inhalant gases used for or in conjunction with injectable euthanasia products can be used for euthanasia. Anesthetic gases such as Isoflurane can be used alone or to induce anesthesia prior to the use of injectable pentobarbital. Because of the toxic nature of pentobarbital animals destine for use as food or food products can be euthanized with gases such as carbon dioxide, nitrogen, argon and carbon monoxide. Although toxic if respired, these gases leave the animal safe for consumption.

Non-inhalants such as barbiturates can provide an overdose and mortality. MS222 (tricaine methane sulfonate) can be used in fish and amphibians to facilitate euthanasia. Potassium chloride is used in conjunction with other euthanasia products, but should not be used by itself.

Physical methods of acceptable euthanasia include the use of a captive bolt, gunshot, cervical dislocation, decapitation, electrocution, microwave irradiation and exsanguinations. These forms of euthanasia are not generally utilized in companion animal medicine, but can be found in research and farm animal situations. Because of the nature of these techniques they should only be performed by qualified personnel.

Owner Grief and Pain

The decision to euthanize a pet can be a difficult and emotional experience for the pet owner. Most pets are thought of as members of the family; their loss is tremendous. Pet owners may be visibly sad and emotional; however they may also be stoic or angry. Faced with these difficult decisions, pet owners may have to elect euthanasia because of financial or logistical reasons. No matter what the emotion, being compassionate is essential. This may not require any words, but may be a sympathetic hand on the shoulder, or the offer of some Kleenex. Owners may request some personal time with the pet prior to and after the pet's death. Some clinics have special rooms available for pet owners to say their goodbyes and regain their composure. Sympathy cards and flower arrangements may be sent by the veterinary practice as a form of condolence.

Post-euthanasia Care of Body

Most veterinary practices have storage facilities for deceased pets; most are in the form of a chest freezer. Freezers enable deceased animals to be stored without becoming spoiled and foul smelling. Trash bags may serve as 'body bags' for deceased pets; this ensures that urine and feces will be contained. Proper identification of the bag is necessary in case the owner would like to collect their pet. Large deceased animals can be difficult to carry; use additional people and a gurney to transport the pet if necessary.

Types of animal disposal include cremation, digestion and rendering. Several crematoriums exist for animals. Incineration is the process by which animals are cremated. Due to EPA emission issues, crematoriums are becoming less prevalent. Tissue digesters are gaining popularity as a means of animal disposal. Tissue digesters use potassium hydroxide (KOH), steam and pressure to dissolve animal tissue. The byproduct of this process is a fertilizer-like material that is safe to the environment. Bones, however, are not completely digested in this process. Rendering facilities utilize animal parts for fertilizers, cosmetics, and animal foods.

Some owners will request that their pet be privately cremated. Cremation and burial companies enable pet owners the opportunity of having a burial plot in a pet cemetery for their pet, or an urn to keep at home.

Also, owners have utilized taxidermy and freezing to preserve their pets for eternity.

The costs of euthanasia services and disposal can be significant. Private cremation and specialty services such as urns and boxes can send euthanasia costs into the hundreds of dollars.

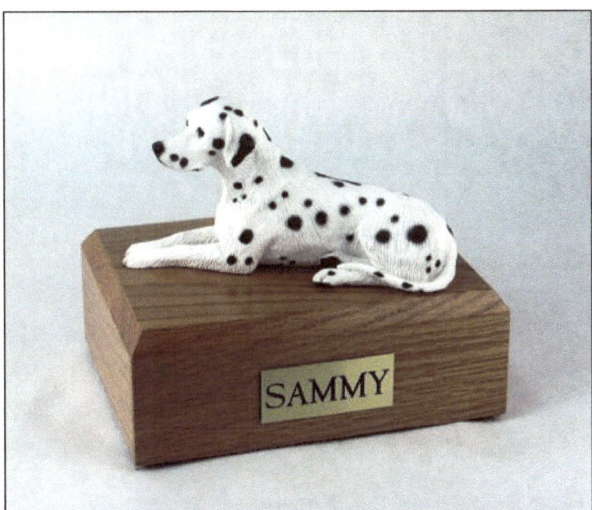

Figure 137: Wood pet urn. For more information go to: www.recover-from-grief.com.

Behavior

Ethology is the scientific study of behavior. Animal behavior is an important tool for the veterinary professional, as this can help recognize behavior types and aid in appropriate handling and care.

Behavior can be broken down into two fundamental types: instinctive behaviors and learned behaviors.

For animals, *instinctive behaviors* include those that are genetically hard-wired such as scent marking and predatory behaviors. The kneading action of the paws of puppies and kittens when nursing is an instinctive behavior.

Learned behaviors are shaped by experience and include social interactions with other animals, some types of aggression and those such as sitting and rolling over that are trained by the owner. Associative learning is the basis of most animal training and can utilize classical or operant conditioning. These training techniques use the association of a sound, object or treat for example, to reinforce a particular behavior. Operant conditioning, furthermore, utilizes several reinforcement types including:

- Positive reinforcement
- Negative reinforcement
- Positive punishment
- Negative punishment

In all of these cases, positive refers to an addition and negative implies a subtraction. Reinforcement refers to a behavior that is increased in frequency and punishment causes the behavior to decrease in frequency.

Positive Reinforcement	A behavior is followed by a rewarding stimulus and the behavior increases. For example, giving a treat to a dog for sitting.
Negative Reinforcement	A behavior is followed by the removal of an adverse stimulus and the behavior increases. For example, the removal of a loud noise when the dog sits.
Positive Punishment	A behavior is followed by a stimulus resulting in the decrease of the behavior. For example, popping a balloon in front of a dog when he barks.
Negative Punishment	A behavior is followed by removal of a stimulus resulting in the decrease of the behavior. For example, taking away a favorite toy when the dog barks.

Table 34: Operant conditioning strategies

Observational learning or modeling occurs as a result of observing and replicating behaviors of another animal.

Animals may recognize your fear before you recognize theirs; animals will take advantage of your fear, therefore be confident when working with them.

Imprinting can occur in the absence of a parent animal. This is common in birds, especially ducks and geese, when a human association is made by the newly hatched chick in the absence of the parent bird.

Animal communication includes visual, auditory and olfactory forms. Dogs and cats have heightened senses of smell and hearing. Dogs are used by law enforcement to locate explosives, drugs and people because of their acute sense of smell. They use these senses to communicate with other animals and people. This communication may include barking (vocalization), body posturing (gestures) or scent marking (olfaction). It is important that veterinary staff recognize and interpret these communication methods utilized by animals.

Behavior problems can be a tremendous problem for some pet owners. Left untreated, aberrant behaviors can result in property damage, pet or human injury or euthanasia of the problematic animal. Many behavioral problems can be remedied with proper training.

Aggression, one of the more common and dangerous behavioral problems, can result from many circumstances; fear is an important form of aggression seen in the veterinary clinic. Fear can lead to bites and injury if not recognized. The use of muzzles and restraint devices for these animals is essential. Aggression can also manifest itself in maternal, hierarchal and sexual situations.

Separation anxiety can lead to property damage, barking and house soiling.

Scent marking, a typically normal animal behavior, can be problematic for the pet owner.

Breeds

All domestic dog breeds are descended from wolves. The desirable hunting characteristics of the wolf led to the domestication of the first dogs over 12,000 years ago. Selective breeding for specific characteristics led to the radiation of dog species; some were bred for speed while others were bred for size, color or other beneficial characteristics. Man's ability to breed for specific characteristics has led to the dog breeds seen today. These breeds are referred to as 'purebred' and are a result of a pairing of two like individuals. Mixed breed dogs, also referred to as mutts, are a result of the breeding of two different breeds of dog. In an attempt to maintain the lineage of purebred dogs, several animal breed organizations were established. In the United States, the American Kennel Club (AKC) was established as a registry of purebred dogs. The AKC currently recognizes seven groups of purebred dogs encompassing over 180 breeds. These groups are as follows:

- Sporting breeds like the Labrador retriever, Pointer and Vizsla.
- Hound breeds like the Greyhound, Beagle and Dachshund.
- Working breeds like the Akita, Doberman pinscher and Rottweiler.
- Terrier breeds like the Bull, Irish and Wire Fox Terriers.
- Toy breeds like the Chihuahua, Maltese and Poodle.
- Non-sporting breeds like the Bulldog, Shar-Pei and Dalmatian.
- Herding breeds like the Australian shepherd, Border collie and Shetland sheepdog.

Of the over 180 purebred dog breeds recognized by the AKC, the most popular is the Labrador retriever, followed by the German shepherd and Yorkshire terrier. It has been suggested that the Border collie is the smartest of all the dog breeds.

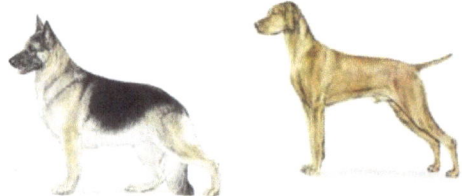

Figure 138: The German shepherd (left), and Vizsla. Thanks to AKC.org

The history of the domestic cat goes back over 5,000 years. Domestic cats have changed little from their wild counterparts. Their ability to be independent and efficient hunters, made them desirable companions and 'pest controllers'. There are nearly 100 purebred breeds of cats. Mixed cat breeds are sometimes referred to by their hair coat length; Domestic longhair or shorthair.

Dog and cat breeding is a topic of debate because of the underlying concern of inbreeding. In an attempt to maintain ideal characteristics for purebred animals, inbreeding has been used. Inbreeding can lead to genetic problems and the perpetuation of genetically based diseases from one generation to the next. Examples include hip dysplasia, patellar luxation and heart disease. It is this concern that has led some people to prefer 'mutts' over purebred dogs and cats.

Genetics

Genetics is the biological science of genes and heredity in living organisms. Genes are found in the DNA of all organisms; the inheritance of these genes is a result of the combination of genetic material from the individual's parents. Gregor Mendel was able to determine with plants, that inheritance could be easily predicted and explained mathematically. Mendel's work enabled scientists to understand the genetic basis of heredity. Dog and cat breeders use genetics to perpetuate desirable traits in their animals. These observed traits, known as phenotypes, are especially important when the animal is being judged in a competition. Breeding two individuals with desirable phenotypes can result in offspring with identical or more desirable characteristics; the genotypes of the individuals are passed to their offspring. These genotypes are even more likely to be perpetuated if they are 'dominant'. Unlike dominant genes, recessive genes are less likely to be seen phenotypically, but in some instances, they too, can be expressed. By using a Punnett square, the mixing of genotypes of two individuals can show the resultant phenotypes and proportion of its occurrence in the individual's offspring. In the first example, two individuals with dominant 'H' genes also known as homozygous, when bred will produce four individuals with the 'HH' phenotype. If the 'H' gene represented long hair, then all of the offspring would have long hair. If however, two individuals that had both a dominant 'H' and a recessive 'h' gene were bred together, genetically, the resultant offspring would have one individual with 'HH', two with 'Hh' and one with 'hh'. If the recessive gene produced short hair, then phenotypically, three of the offspring would have long hair and one would have short hair. Because the 'H' is dominant, the individuals with the 'Hh' genotype, also known as heterozygous, would have long hair in spite of having the recessive gene present.

	H	H
H	HH	HH
H	HH	HH

Table 35: Punnett square showing a combination of genes with two homozygous individuals

	H	h
H	HH	Hh
h	Hh	hh

Table 36: Punnett square showing a combination of genes with two heterozygous individuals

A lot of genes are found on the chromosomes common to both male and female organisms; these are called autosomal chromosomes. A few genes, however, are located on the chromosomes that determine an organism's gender; these are called the sex-linked chromosomes. Most mammals have the same sex determination system; females have two identical chromosomes (XX), and males have two distinctly different chromosomes (XY). An example of a sex-linked trait is the calico cat, which is almost always a female. Calico cats are domestic cats with spotted coats of primarily white with orange and black patches. The X chromosome determines the color of a cat and since the male only has one X chromosome he cannot have both orange and non-orange coloration.

Sickle cell anemia, hemophilia and Down's syndrome are examples of genetically manifested diseases seen in humans.

Office Procedures

Veterinary practices usually have a client and patient receiving and waiting area. This area may be designed so cats and dogs are separated from each other or provide barriers for client privacy. The floors are generally non-carpeted in the event an 'accident' occurs. The waiting area is where the client first interacts with the receptionist. The receptionist is generally in charge of greeting and checking in the client and patient. Other duties include answering phones, filing records and collecting fees for services.

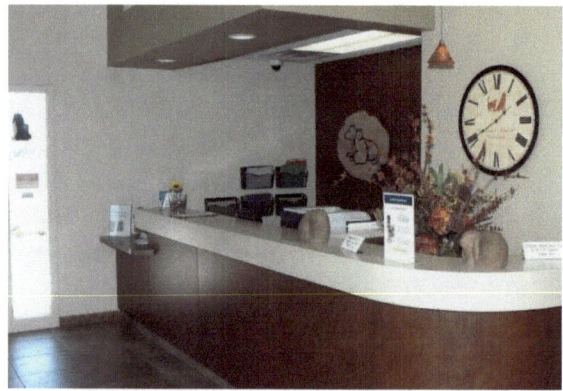

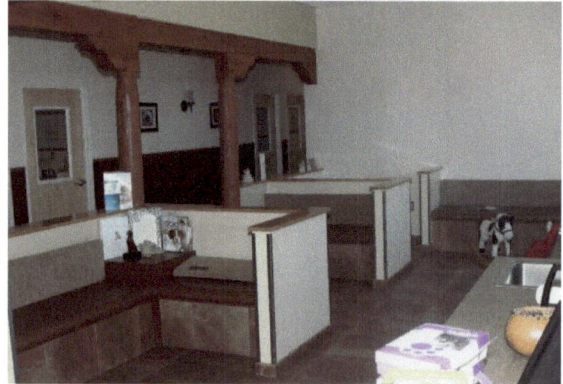

Figure 139: Reception desk and waiting room

Interacting with clients while answering phones can be an overwhelming task; many clinics also have multiple phone lines making the job more challenging. When answering the phone, one should be courteous and articulate, as the person you are talking to may be a potential client. If it is necessary to place a client on hold, ask them if they are experiencing an emergency or if they would be willing to be put on hold; this is a simple way to show them how important they are to you and the clinic.

Communication is an important aspect of the veterinary professionals' daily life. Effective communication with clients and coworkers is necessary in most jobs, but especially in veterinary medicine. Clients can be sad or angry; calm effective communication can diffuse these difficult situations.
It can be argued that group dynamics are more important than job skills. Employees who have positive attitudes can be easily trained to do their job; employees who argue and don't get along create tension and a toxic work environment. A positive attitude can create great client relations and bolster employee work quality.

Sexual harassment should never be tolerated by anyone. It is defined as unwelcome verbal, visual or physical conduct of a sexual nature. Identifying and managing sexual harassment has become more common in the workplace; punishment for these behaviors can be substantial. It is important to review and follow all clinic policies regarding etiquette and harassment to ensure violations are not occurring.
Office duties are an essential component to a successful veterinary practice. Computers have made office procedures, such as scheduling patients and billing much more efficient. Basic knowledge of computers is important for all members of the veterinary team.

Conclusion

By now you should have read these pages, memorized the terminology and learned some new concepts. You have hopefully recognized that the anatomy and physiology of the dog and cat differs little from your own, making it easier to understand how the body functions. You have begun to understand medical math and are less fearful of the metric system. You understand the importance of proper health, safety and restraint techniques to prevent personal injury or injury to others, including the pet. You now look at a dog and see more than just a cute furry animal that loves to play with squeaky toys. Together, all of these things have given you the most valuable tool of all; confidence. Use this confidence when interviewing for a veterinary job, when restraining a patient in the exam room and when talking to clients about vaccines and other topics. Your confidence will impress potential employers, clients and will be recognized by the animal patients you work with; this aspect you will find to be of the utmost importance.

So, What Do You Do Now?

1. Create a resume. Make it simple in design; be concise. Try and limit your resume to a single page. Use animal and leadership experiences in your resume. Always dress for success in an interview.
2. If you don't already have one, get a medical encyclopedia. You will be exposed to more medical terms in your career; if you do not know a word, look it up!
3. Get a good quality stethoscope. It will make a huge difference. It need not be the most expensive one, but don't get a cheap one. Go to MyVetEssentials.com for the one I prefer.
4. Many small animal veterinary practices are beginning to see exotic animals, i.e. birds, reptiles and rodents. Learn about these unique animals. Go to MyVetEssentials.com for The Veterinary Assisting Essential Book of Knowledge-Exotics.
5. Enjoy the ever changing world of veterinary medicine; pursue your passion. If you truly enjoy your job, then it will never be work.

Confidence is the key, be confident in all things you do; never hesitate.